THE
BRAIN
FITNESS
BOOK

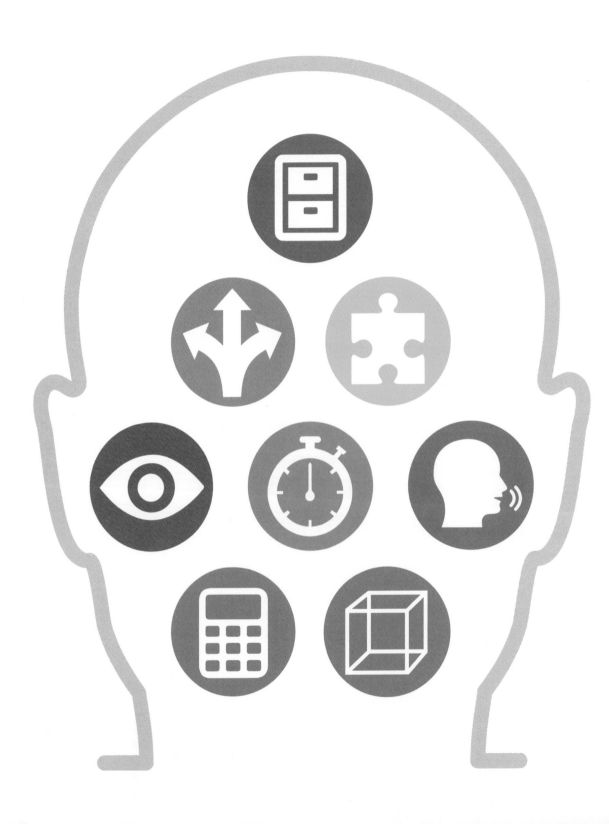

THE
BRAIN
FITNESS
BOOK

Activities and puzzles
to keep your mind active and healthy

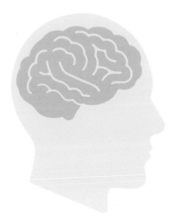

RITA CARTER

CONTENTS

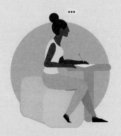

⑧ HOW THE BRAIN WORKS

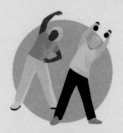

㉖ BRAIN WORKOUT

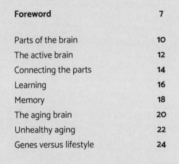

DK Penguin Random House

DK LONDON

Senior Editor
Rob Houston

Project Editor
Miezan van Zyl

Editors
Claire Gell, Wendy Horobin,
Victoria Pyke

US Editor
Margaret Parrish

Executive US Editor
Lori Hand

Senior Production Controller
Meskerem Berhane

Managing Editor
Angeles Gavira Guerrero

Associate Publishing Director
Liz Wheeler

Publishing Director
Jonathan Metcalf

Project Art Editor
Francis Wong

Designers
Sunita Gahir, Shahid Mahmood

Illustrators
Mark Clifton, Sunita Gahir,
Phil Gamble, Edwood Burn

**Jacket Design
Development Manager**
Sophia MTT

Jacket Designer
Stephanie Cheng Hui Tan

Production Editor
Kavita Varma

Managing Art Editor
Michael Duffy

Art Director
Karen Self

DK INDIA

Senior Managing Editor
Rohan Sinha

Jacket Designer
Priyanka Bansal

Picture Researcher
Surya Sarangi

Picture Research Manager
Taiyaba Khatoon

Production Manager
Pankaj Sharma

Editorial head
Glenda Fernandes

Managing Art Editor
Sudakshina Basu

Project Art Editor
Rupanki Arora Kaushik

Art Editors
Rabia Ahmad, Debjyoti Mukherjee

Assistant Art Editor
Aarushi Dhawan

DTP Designers
Anita Yadav, Nand Kishor Acharya

Pre-production Manager
Balwant Singh

Design head
Malavika Talukder

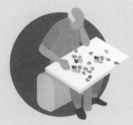

(50)
THINKING SKILLS

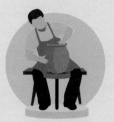

(78)
TRY NEW THINGS

First American Edition, 2021
Published in the United States by DK Publishing
1450 Broadway, Suite 801, New York, NY 10018

Copyright © 2021 Dorling Kindersley Limited
DK, a Division of Penguin Random House LLC
21 22 23 24 25 10 9 8 7 6 5 4 3 2 1
001–322043–Apr/2021

A catalog record for this book
is available from the Library of Congress.
ISBN 978-0-7440-2837-9

DK books are available at special discounts when purchased in bulk for sales promotions, premiums, fund-raising, or educational use. For details, contact:
DK Publishing Special Markets, 1450 Broadway, Suite 801, New York, NY 10018
SpecialSales@dk.com

Printed and bound in China

For the curious
www.dk.com

Author **RITA CARTER**

Rita Carter writes, broadcasts, and lectures about the human brain. She is the author of the globally successful *Mapping the Mind*, *Exploring Consciousness*, and Dorling Kinderley's *The Brain Book*, among others. Rita has won many prizes for her writing and was awarded a Ph.D from Leuven University for her contribution to brain science.

Puzzle creator **DR. GARETH MOORE**

Dr. Gareth Moore is the author of many puzzle books for children and adults. He is the creator of www.BrainedUp.com and runs the daily puzzle website www.PuzzleMix.com. He earned his Ph.D from Cambridge University (UK) in the field of Machine Learning.

READER NOTICE

While the information in this book has been carefully researched, the publisher and author are not engaged in providing health and fitness advice for individual readers. The information in this book is therefore not a substitute for expert advice and cannot replace sound judgment and good decision-making in matters relating to personal health and fitness. Physical activities are potentially hazardous and the scope of this book does not allow for disclosure of all the risks involved in such activities. If you have any health problems or medical conditions, you are advised always to consult a doctor or other health professional for specific information on such matters. Do not try to self-diagnose or self-treat serious or long-term problems without first consulting a qualified medical practitioner as appropriate, and always seek professional medical advice if problems persist. If you are pregnant or taking prescribed medicines, seek medical advice before changing, stopping, or starting any medical treatment or using any supplements or alternative therapy. Never disregard expert medical advice or delay in seeking advice or treatment due to information obtained from this book. Neither the publisher nor the authors can accept any liability for loss, injury, or damage arising directly or indirectly from any use or misuse of information and advice in this book.

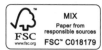

MIX
Paper from responsible sources
FSC™ C018179

This book was made with Forest Stewardship Council™ certified paper—one small step in DK's commitment to a sustainable future. For more information go to www.dk.com/our-green-pledge

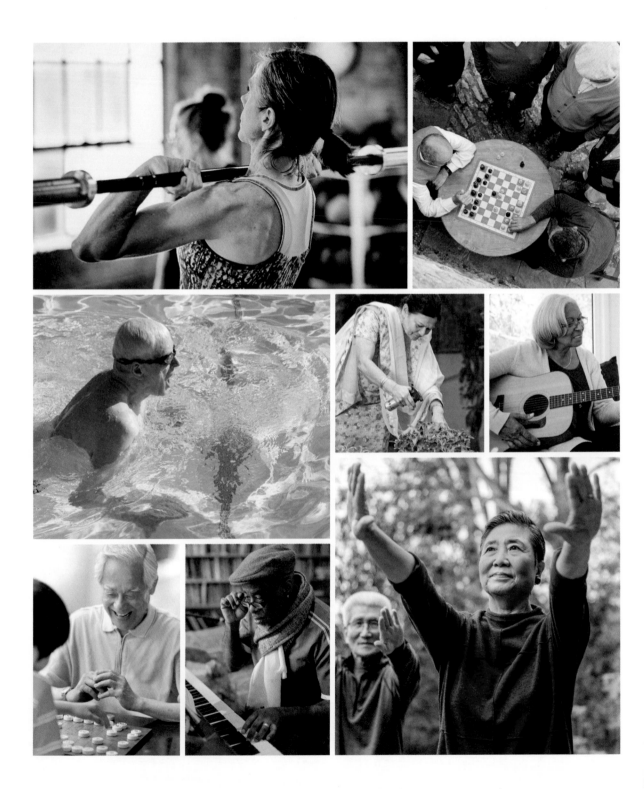

FOREWORD

**YOUR MIND IS ONLY AS GOOD AS THE BRAIN
THAT PRODUCES IT.**

Your memory of a sunny day in childhood, the smell of jasmine, your ability to find your car keys, read the newspaper, and cook a meal all depend on maintaining a well-functioning brain. It is the most important part of your body, because it generates all your experience and controls everything you do.

Despite this, the enormous importance of keeping your brain fit and healthy is generally overlooked. We are bombarded with advice on how to keep our hearts and muscles in order, but information about the best way to preserve our cognitive faculties usually goes no further than the suggestion that we do occasional crosswords.

This book is designed to fill that gap. It pulls together some of the latest scientific research on brain health and shows you how best to achieve it in youth, maintain it through midlife, and preserve and perhaps enhance it in later years.

First, it reveals the complex physical processes that produce thoughts, perceptions, and feelings. Then it explains how you can support, and perhaps enhance these processes. This includes the exercises and nutrition now shown to be especially good for the brain, and advice on how to help prevent or cope with common brain disorders such as stroke and dementia.

The Brain Fitness Book describes the variety of mental skills that work together to produce a fully functioning mind and how each of them can be honed, exercised, and refined to make their best contribution. You can test these skills to explore your own strengths and weaknesses.

Finally, *The Brain Fitness Book* provides a catalog of activities from which you can pick 'n mix to find a brain-healthy lifestyle filled with newly discovered interests. It includes practical guidance to help and encourage you to get started on the activities of your choice.

Rita Carter

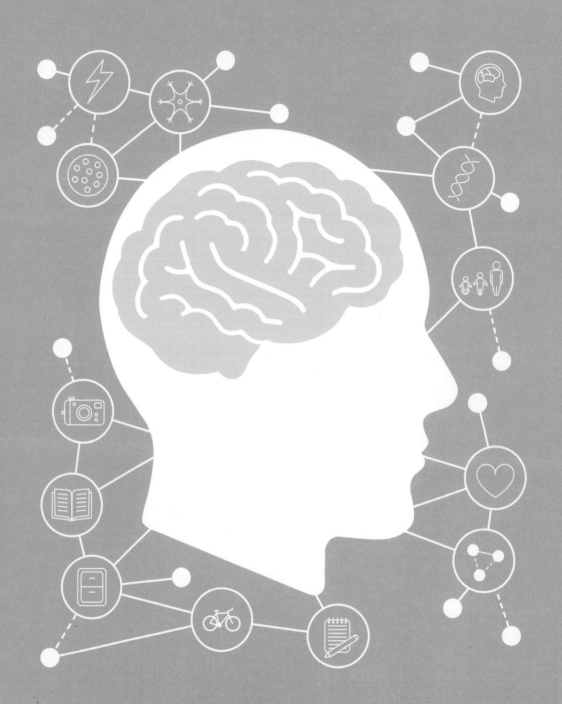

HOW
THE BRAIN
WORKS

PARTS OF THE BRAIN

Your brain is made up of hundreds of modules, each of which does something slightly different. Together, they produce everything you think of as your mind—your perceptions, memories, judgments, and thoughts—and conduct the countless processes that control your body.

THREE-LAYER BRAIN

The brain is made up of three major layers; the oldest layer is at the bottom and the most recently evolved is at the top. At the base is the brain stem, which deals with basic survival. Above the brain stem is the limbic system, which generates emotions. On the top is the cerebrum. Its outer layer is called the cortex, and this produces conscious thought, perceptions, and judgment.

HALF SLICE VIEW
This brain has been sliced in half lengthwise. Half of the limbic system and brain stem are revealed, under the cerebrum's right hemisphere.

SPECIALIZED AREAS
While the cerebrum can be separated into lobes, its outer layer—the cortex—can be mapped more precisely according to functions that occur in specific areas. Deeper brain structures can also be identified with specific tasks.

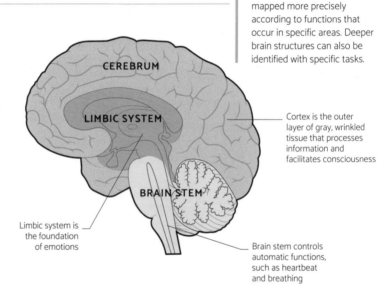

CEREBRUM

LIMBIC SYSTEM

BRAIN STEM

Cortex is the outer layer of gray, wrinkled tissue that processes information and facilitates consciousness

Limbic system is the foundation of emotions

Brain stem controls automatic functions, such as heartbeat and breathing

THE CEREBRAL LOBES

The cerebrum is made of two hemispheres, left and right. Each hemisphere consists of four main lobes divided by deep grooves. Each lobe deals with a different type of function.

LEFT HEMISPHERE
This view shows the whole brain from the left side. This is the brain's left hemisphere, showing the outer surface of the cerebrum—the cortex.

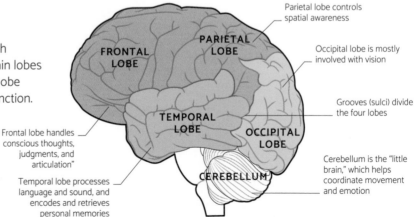

Parietal lobe controls spatial awareness

PARIETAL LOBE

FRONTAL LOBE

Occipital lobe is mostly involved with vision

Grooves (sulci) divide the four lobes

TEMPORAL LOBE

OCCIPITAL LOBE

CEREBELLUM

Frontal lobe handles conscious thoughts, judgments, and articulation"

Temporal lobe processes language and sound, and encodes and retrieves personal memories

Cerebellum is the "little brain," which helps coordinate movement and emotion

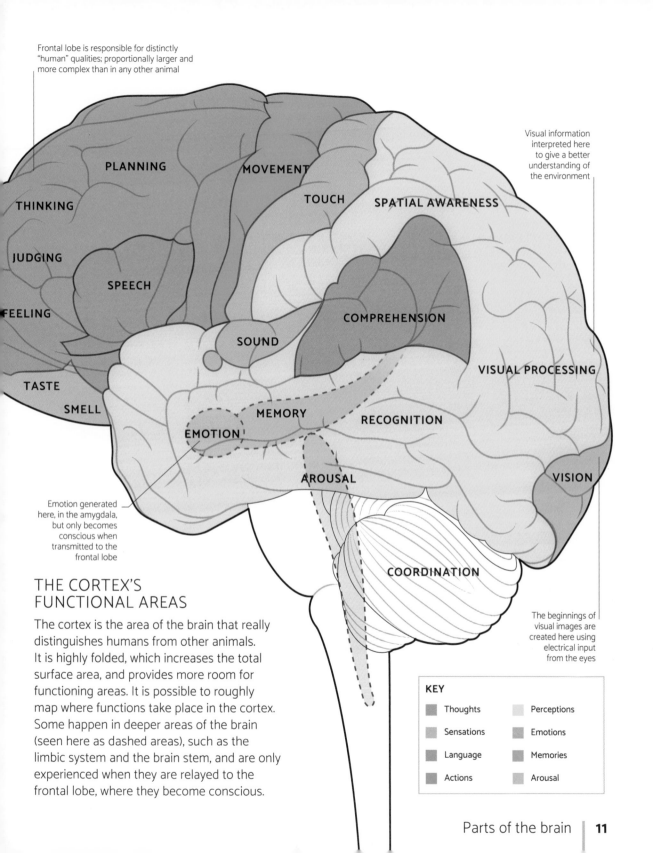

Frontal lobe is responsible for distinctly "human" qualities; proportionally larger and more complex than in any other animal

PLANNING

MOVEMENT

THINKING

TOUCH

SPATIAL AWARENESS

Visual information interpreted here to give a better understanding of the environment

JUDGING

SPEECH

FEELING

COMPREHENSION

SOUND

TASTE

VISUAL PROCESSING

SMELL

MEMORY

RECOGNITION

EMOTION

AROUSAL

VISION

Emotion generated here, in the amygdala, but only becomes conscious when transmitted to the frontal lobe

COORDINATION

THE CORTEX'S FUNCTIONAL AREAS

The cortex is the area of the brain that really distinguishes humans from other animals. It is highly folded, which increases the total surface area, and provides more room for functioning areas. It is possible to roughly map where functions take place in the cortex. Some happen in deeper areas of the brain (seen here as dashed areas), such as the limbic system and the brain stem, and are only experienced when they are relayed to the frontal lobe, where they become conscious.

The beginnings of visual images are created here using electrical input from the eyes

KEY

- Thoughts
- Sensations
- Language
- Actions
- Perceptions
- Emotions
- Memories
- Arousal

THE ACTIVE BRAIN

To keep your brain healthy you need to maintain both its structure–the actual flesh–and the flow of electrical signals that make it work.

FUELING THE BRAIN

A dense web of arteries carries blood to the brain's cells, supplying them with the oxygen and glucose they need to function. The brain cannot store glucose, and so needs a constant supply, and it can only last a few minutes without oxygen before irreparable damage is caused.

BRAIN ARTERIES
The complex webbed arrangement of the brain's arteries allows blood to be supplied by another route if one becomes blocked.

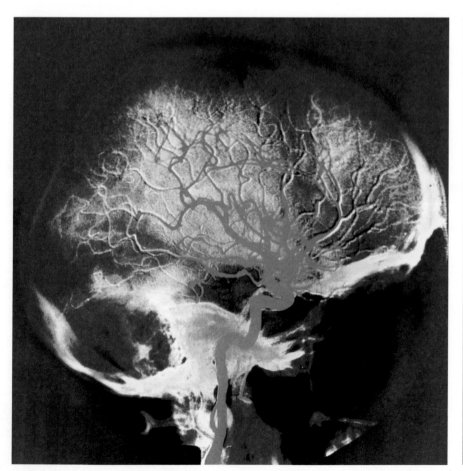

CEREBROSPINAL FLUID (CSF)

Small cavities in the brain called ventricles have special cell linings that produce CSF–a liquid that constantly circulates through the brain. CSF washes away the breakdown products of brain metabolism–a vital job that helps to keep the brain free of the buildup of waste matter.

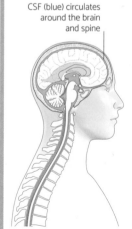

CSF (blue) circulates around the brain and spine

SENDING MESSAGES

Throughout the brain are trillions of electrical cells called neurons, which transmit signals. Each neuron has a single axon, a biological "wire," that carries the signals quickly from one end to the other. A tissue called myelin insulates the axons and this is what makes up the brain's white matter. When two neurons "talk" frequently, the axon from the first will grow toward the other. Growing axons increase the density of the brain. Most neurons are separated by tiny gaps called synapses. A neuron "talks" to the next neuron by transmitting its signal over the synapse using chemicals called neurotransmitters.

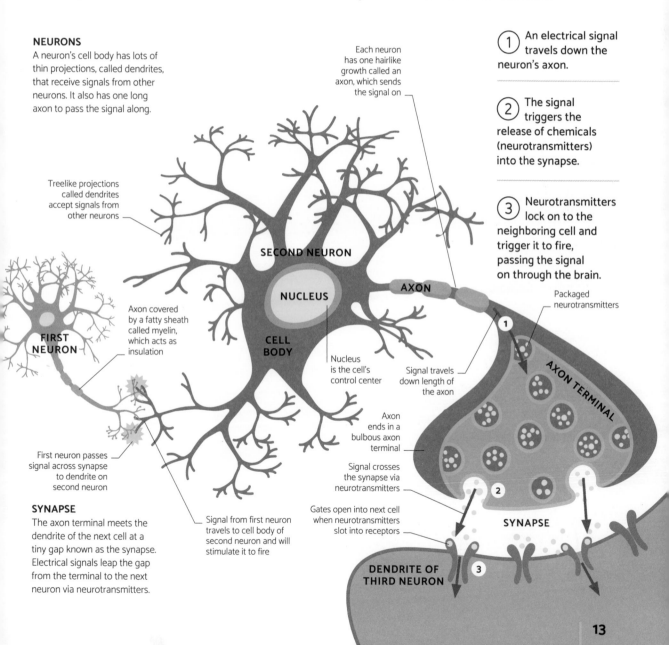

NEURONS
A neuron's cell body has lots of thin projections, called dendrites, that receive signals from other neurons. It also has one long axon to pass the signal along.

Each neuron has one hairlike growth called an axon, which sends the signal on

(1) An electrical signal travels down the neuron's axon.

(2) The signal triggers the release of chemicals (neurotransmitters) into the synapse.

(3) Neurotransmitters lock on to the neighboring cell and trigger it to fire, passing the signal on through the brain.

Treelike projections called dendrites accept signals from other neurons

SECOND NEURON

NUCLEUS

AXON

Packaged neurotransmitters

Axon covered by a fatty sheath called myelin, which acts as insulation

FIRST NEURON

CELL BODY

Nucleus is the cell's control center

Signal travels down length of the axon

AXON TERMINAL

Axon ends in a bulbous axon terminal

First neuron passes signal across synapse to dendrite on second neuron

Signal crosses the synapse via neurotransmitters

SYNAPSE
The axon terminal meets the dendrite of the next cell at a tiny gap known as the synapse. Electrical signals leap the gap from the terminal to the next neuron via neurotransmitters.

Signal from first neuron travels to cell body of second neuron and will stimulate it to fire

Gates open into next cell when neurotransmitters slot into receptors

SYNAPSE

DENDRITE OF THIRD NEURON

CONNECTING THE PARTS

The brain's parts are densely connected so that they work as a single system. Signals travel through the gray matter (nerve cell bodies), as well as to and from the underlying areas.

THE BRAIN'S WIRING

The connections between neurons form the "wiring" of the brain. Bundles of nerve cell fibers, or axons (see p.13), fan out to connect to all parts of the cortex. The axons are wrapped in fatty material and form the brain's "white matter." The pattern of neural pathways is similar in all of us, but differs in detail from person to person.

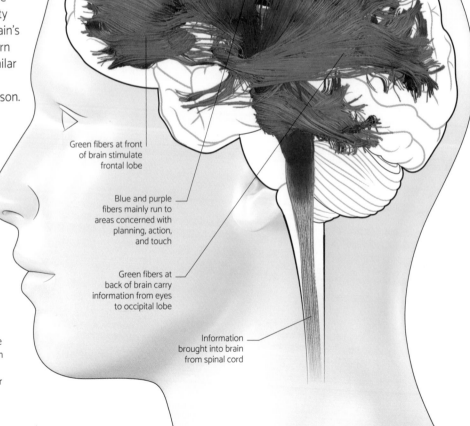

Green fibers at front of brain stimulate frontal lobe

Blue and purple fibers mainly run to areas concerned with planning, action, and touch

Green fibers at back of brain carry information from eyes to occipital lobe

Information brought into brain from spinal cord

NERVE PATHWAYS
A global initiative called the Connectome Project charts the brain's neural pathways using a form of MRI (magnetic resonance imaging) scanning called diffusion tensor imaging. The resulting pictures colour code white matter with rainbow hues.

THE BRAIN STEM

The brain's nerve tracts do not end at the neck; they extend right through your body–sending and receiving information. The bridge between the cortex (the higher brain) and the rest of the nervous system is the brain stem. The brain stem controls automatic functions and many aspects of attention.

THE LIMBIC SYSTEM

Instinctive drives such as aggression, fear, and appetite are handled by the limbic system, along with some movement, learning, memory, and higher mental activities. Nerve axons link all of its parts.

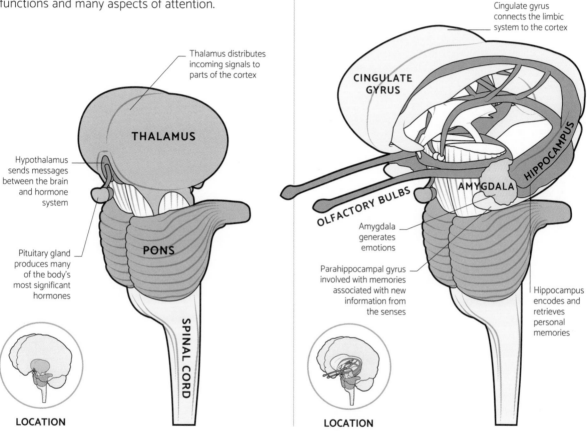

Thalamus distributes incoming signals to parts of the cortex

THALAMUS

Hypothalamus sends messages between the brain and hormone system

Pituitary gland produces many of the body's most significant hormones

PONS

SPINAL CORD

LOCATION

Cingulate gyrus connects the limbic system to the cortex

CINGULATE GYRUS

HIPPOCAMPUS

OLFACTORY BULBS

AMYGDALA

Amygdala generates emotions

Parahippocampal gyrus involved with memories associated with new information from the senses

Hippocampus encodes and retrieves personal memories

LOCATION

SIGNAL LAYERS

The brain's wrinkled surface (the cortex) mostly consists of six layers of tissue containing different types of neurons. Information from the lower parts of the brain feed up to the cortex and may then be passed sideways along it, up or down to another layer, or back down to the lower part. This electrical signaling generates our conscious experience.

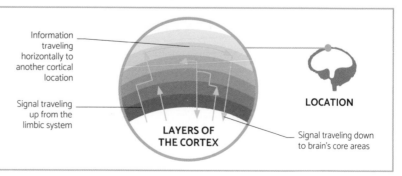

Information traveling horizontally to another cortical location

Signal traveling up from the limbic system

LAYERS OF THE CORTEX

LOCATION

Signal traveling down to brain's core areas

LEARNING

Every bit of knowledge–each fact, skill, face, tune, place: anything you can say you "know,"–is stored in the brain as a unique network of electrically linked cells. Learning involves creating new networks.

Experiences are generated by neurons firing together. Each aspect of an experience is created by active neurons in specific brain areas

REPEATING SIGNALS

Neurons communicate by sending electrical signals (see p.13). Constant chatter between neurons causes them to link up to form a network. If the same neurons fire together often, they eventually become permanently sensitized to each other, so that if one fires, the others do as well.

① If someone sees a red table, the perception is created by neurons firing in the color and shape areas of the brain. It is first perceived as something red and square.

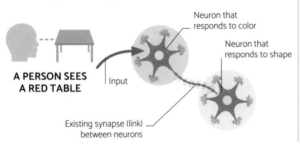

A PERSON SEES A RED TABLE

Input

Neuron that responds to color

Neuron that responds to shape

Existing synapse (link) between neurons

② As the shape and color neurons fire, the person recognizes the object as a table, so "table" recognizing neurons fire. A third group of neurons therefore get joined up.

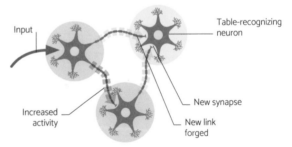

Input

Table-recognizing neuron

Increased activity

New synapse

New link forged

③ The three neuron groups continue to fire together and become linked in a network, forming the memory of the table.

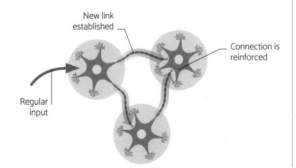

New link established

Connection is reinforced

Regular input

④ If the person notes that the table is on their right, the "position" sending neurons fire and join up to make "red, square, table to my right."

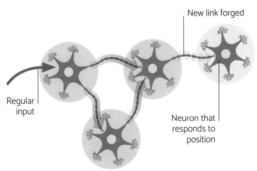

New link forged

Regular input

Neuron that responds to position

EXPERT NETWORKS

Different aspects of things stimulate different areas of the brain. When the active cells in the stimulated areas join up, they form a network that represents an item of knowledge. People who learn a great deal about a particular thing, or develop extraordinary expertise, may develop localized increases in brain density. One famous study used brain-imaging technology to examine the brains of London taxi drivers. The subjects were found to have measurably more tissue in the route-finding area of the brain.

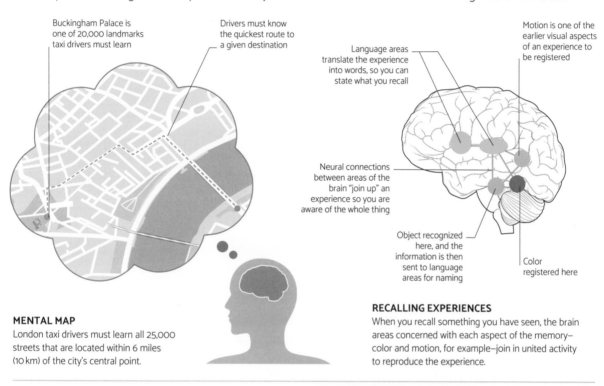

Buckingham Palace is one of 20,000 landmarks taxi drivers must learn

Drivers must know the quickest route to a given destination

Language areas translate the experience into words, so you can state what you recall

Motion is one of the earlier visual aspects of an experience to be registered

Neural connections between areas of the brain "join up" an experience so you are aware of the whole thing

Object recognized here, and the information is then sent to language areas for naming

Color registered here

MENTAL MAP
London taxi drivers must learn all 25,000 streets that are located within 6 miles (10 km) of the city's central point.

RECALLING EXPERIENCES
When you recall something you have seen, the brain areas concerned with each aspect of the memory—color and motion, for example—join in united activity to reproduce the experience.

GROWING NEURONS

New neurons are made in the human brain, a process known as neurogenesis, throughout life. Once they are formed, the new cells integrate with older neurons. Neurogenesis is thought to help preserve knowledge and possibly enhance certain types of learning. In mice, physical activity and mental stimulation have been found to increase neurogenesis.

NEUROGENESIS
New nerve cells can be encouraged to form in a lab. This micrograph shows new neural cells during a stage where they can specialize into either neurons or support cells.

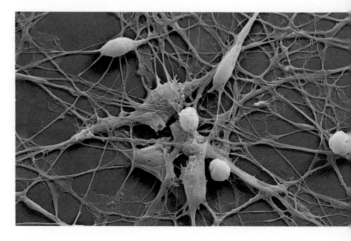

MEMORY

Many of our everyday experiences pass through
our brain and are not stored, but some experiences
and information are encoded in our brain as memories.
The purpose of retaining experiences of the past is to
help us navigate experiences in the present.

**The human
brain starts
remembering
things while
in the womb**

WORKING MEMORY

There are several different types
of memory (see p.19), each of
which uses a different set of brain
areas; this also means one type
may be poor, while another is
excellent. Working memory is the
ability to hold information in mind
just long enough to use it, and
it involves activation of brain
regions in both the left and right
hemispheres. Here, they are
shown working together to keep
an item of information in mind.

Central executive area
holds entire plan,
including language

Broca's area is used
as "inner voice" that
repeats information

Auditory and language
area maintains sound of
item to be remembered

**CENTRAL
EXECUTIVE
AREA**

**BROCA'S
AREA**

**AUDITORY
AND LANGUAGE
AREA**

Areas continue to
activate each other in
a loop until attention
is withdrawn

**The inability
of most adults
to recall
memories
from before
the of age 4 is
called infantile
amnesia**

LEFT HEMISPHERE
For most people, the left
hemisphere contains language
areas that activate the sounds of
the words to be remembered, a
phone number, for example.

WHY DO WE FORGET?

Memories fade when the network of neurons that encodes them disintegrates. If we do not frequently reuse and strengthen a network in our long-term memory we may be unable to access that information, although it may still remain "stored." Some forgetting is normal, but forgetting becomes a problem if the brain's networks decay prematurely.

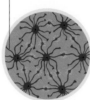

Long-term memories stored as networks of connections

If a memory is not recalled for years, many connections will be lost

FORGETTING
Recalling a memory activates it, strengthening the synapses, but without reactivation, connections will not be strengthened.

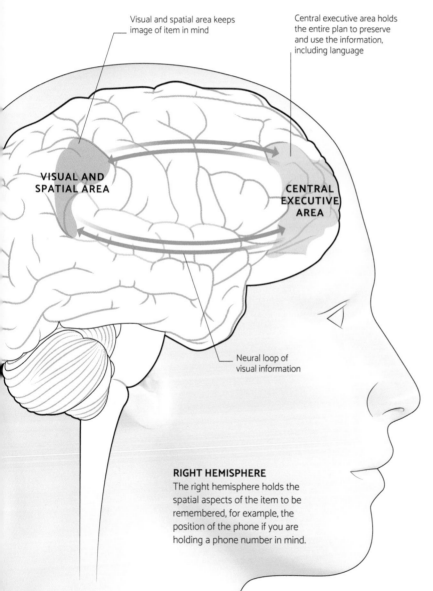

Visual and spatial area keeps image of item in mind

Central executive area holds the entire plan to preserve and use the information, including language

VISUAL AND SPATIAL AREA

CENTRAL EXECUTIVE AREA

Neural loop of visual information

RIGHT HEMISPHERE
The right hemisphere holds the spatial aspects of the item to be remembered, for example, the position of the phone if you are holding a phone number in mind.

TYPES OF MEMORY

EPISODIC MEMORY
Recalling events that were personally experienced, a wedding day, for instance. Parts of the brain involved depends on the experience.

SEMANTIC MEMORY
Recalling things you know, for example, that the capital of France is Paris. Facts are recalled from the temporal lobe (see p.10).

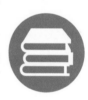

PROCEDURAL MEMORY
Recalling motor actions that are now automatic, such as riding a bike. These skills are stored in brain areas that lie beneath the cortex.

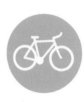

WORKING MEMORY
Remembering something just long enough to use it, for example, keeping a phone number in mind until you have dialed it (see left).

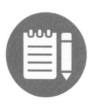

THE AGING BRAIN

Like any other organ, the brain changes with time, and some of the changes make it less efficient. Unlike most other organs, though, the brain is extraordinarily "plastic"; learning and activity can alter its physical structure in ways that make up for the "bad" changes.

Brain volume decreases by 5–10 percent from the age of 20 to 90

COMPENSATING FOR CHANGE

Physical brain changes make cognitive tasks more difficult for older people, who naturally compensate by using more brainpower to achieve the same effect. This may mean that after a hard "thinking" day an older person will feel more tired. Hard work is especially good for the brain; it builds white matter, strengthening and reinforcing the connections between neurons throughout the brain. Older people, therefore, may have more to draw on when looking for a solution to a problem. People who achieve hard-won expertise often reach their peak when they are older, and vocabulary and language skills go on improving throughout life (see p.54).

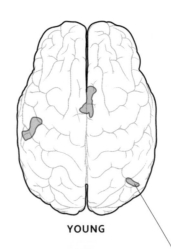
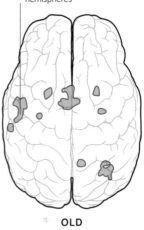

Brain activity in older people is more distributed across both hemispheres

YOUNG

OLD

BRAIN ACTIVATION
A brain-imaging study examined how much brain activation (blue areas) happened when young and old people engaged in physical coordination tasks.

Much less activity, especially in right hemisphere

HAPPINESS LEVELS

A study found that younger and older people reported higher levels of well-being than people who were in middle age. When the results of the study were plotted on a graph it created a U-shape. Happiness levels appear to dip as people enter into their 40s and early 50s, and then rise again. People around age 65 were found to have the same life satisfaction as those in their 20s.

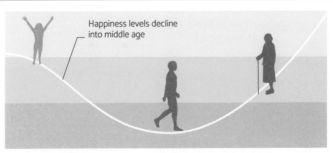

Happiness levels decline into middle age

WELL-BEING

AGE

SHRINKING BRAIN

The human brain loses volume as it ages. The areas affected include the neocortex, which is responsible for thinking; frontal areas concerned with judgment; and limbic areas concerned with memory and emotion. Blood supply diminishes and there are changes in hormones, neurotransmitters, and other chemicals that the brain uses to function. All this tends to slow the brain down and creates problems with memory and coordination. Myelin—the insulation around the signaling part of neurons—breaks down, making signal transmission slower and less reliable. Sometimes "wires" may get crossed.

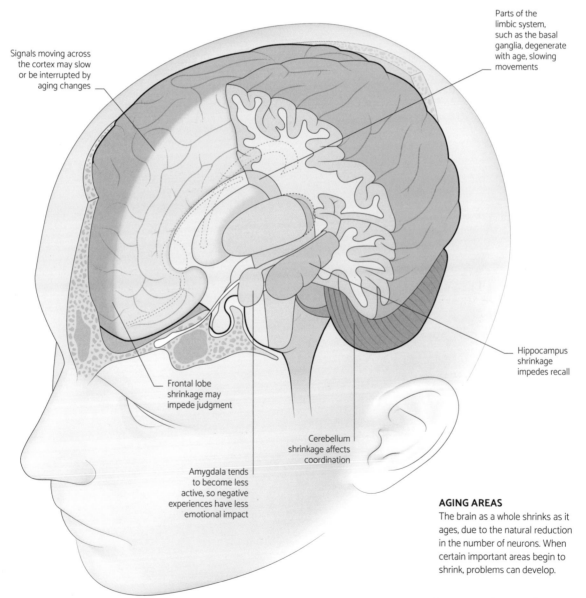

Signals moving across the cortex may slow or be interrupted by aging changes

Parts of the limbic system, such as the basal ganglia, degenerate with age, slowing movements

Frontal lobe shrinkage may impede judgment

Hippocampus shrinkage impedes recall

Amygdala tends to become less active, so negative experiences have less emotional impact

Cerebellum shrinkage affects coordination

AGING AREAS
The brain as a whole shrinks as it ages, due to the natural reduction in the number of neurons. When certain important areas begin to shrink, problems can develop.

UNHEALTHY AGING

If you keep your brain fit, it may serve you well throughout your life. As your brain ages, however, it becomes more susceptible to certain diseases, especially dementia and stroke. Their damage can be seen on a brain scan, but the symptoms are changes in behavior, personality, and mental and physical ability.

Dementia that develops before the age of 65 is known "early-onset dementia"

DEMENTIA

Diseases that kill off brain cells causing early and severe cognitive decline are known in general as dementia. Dementia damages the brain's neurons, which means that the usual messages cannot be sent around the brain as well as normal, and this hinders the body from functioning normally.

ALZHEIMER'S DISEASE

Alzheimer's is a disease marked by progressive decay of brain cells, which causes universal cognitive decline. Diagnosis is usually by behavioral testing, but brain scans can detect the buildup of waste protein, which is thought to cause it.

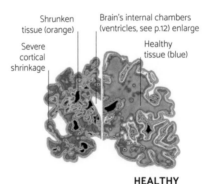

Shrunken tissue (orange)

Severe cortical shrinkage

Brain's internal chambers (ventricles, see p.12) enlarge

Healthy tissue (blue)

ALZHEIMER'S

HEALTHY BRAIN

PARKINSON'S DISEASE

Loss of neurons in the substantia nigra (a part of the brain involved mainly in movement) causes Parkinson's. The brain becomes unable to make enough dopamine to control movement. Drugs and electrical treatment can help manage the condition.

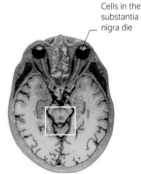

Cells in the substantia nigra die

PARKINSON'S

STROKE

A stroke is caused by a blockage or a bleed in the brain that prevents blood from reaching part of it. A stroke damages or kills a cluster of brain cells.

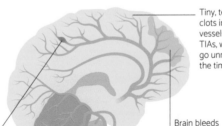

Tiny, temporary clots in blood vessels cause TIAs, which may go unnoticed at the time

TRANSIENT ISCHEMIC ATTACK (TIA)

A TIA is a "mini-stroke" in which a blood clot temporarily starves a part of the brain before breaking up. Symptoms may be subtle, but TIAs tend to recur, and over time they may damage the brain in a similar way to other dementias.

Blood clots in larger blood vessels cause strokes, which damage brain tissue

Brain bleeds may damage large clusters of brain cells, causing memory loss or partial paralysis

AM I AT RISK?

Stroke is a form of cardiovascular disease and it is caused by the same things that cause heart attacks. This means, generally, that those most at risk are people who eat too much junk food, smoke, or don't do much exercise. Alzheimer's disease shares risk factors with stroke, but there is still much that is unknown about why some people get it and others don't. Healthy, age-related brain changes (see pp.20–21) also include loss or deterioration of tissue. People who keep physically healthy and mentally active show less decline and these activities may also make them less vulnerable to disease.

FUNNY "TURNS"

See your doctor if you have a "turn" that involves loss of consciousness, dizziness, or momentary amnesia. TIAs or "mini strokes" (see previous page) may have very subtle and short-lived effects, but if you have one, your risk of having more, or having a major stroke, increases.

BALANCED LIFESTYLE

In addition to natural aging, there are many factors that can increase your risk of stroke or dementia. However, there are also everyday ways to keep your brain as healthy as possible.

RISK OF DISEASE

DELAYS DISEASE

JUNK FOOD

Eating too much fatty food can lead to high cholesterol, which increases your risk of stroke

SMOKING

Smoking has been linked with damage to the brain's cortex and can increase the risk of stroke

NOT ENOUGH EXERCISE

Sitting for long periods and being inactive can increase the risk of brain disease

GETTING OLD

Simply getting older increases your risk; your arteries may also naturally become narrower

MENTAL ACTIVITY

Regularly engaging your brain can build and maintain brain tissue

HEALTHY DIET

Foods such as fresh fruits and whole grains supply vital nutrients for the brain

EXCERCISE

Aerobic exercise keeps your brain well supplied with oxygen and nutrients

GENES VERSUS LIFESTYLE

Genes mold our brains and, although practically every aspect of cognition can be improved and maintained by lifestyle practices, "good" genes make brain fitness easier to achieve.

HEALTH FACTORS
Our genes govern the way our bodies develop and function, but they work in combination with environmental factors to shape us throughout our lives.

GENES AND ENVIRONMENT

Brain health is determined by a complicated interaction between environment and genes. At least 160 genes are directly involved in determining how much a person's brain will shrink with age. Although nearly everyone inherits the same number of genes, the genes themselves vary from person to person, and the variant you inherit affects how things like nutrition and exercise affect your body. Two different people could, therefore, have identical fitness regimes but see quite different outcomes. Experiences you have can also cause chemical changes in your DNA that may stop genes from being activated (see epigenetics, opposite). Scientists can only say what is likely to enhance your health.

CHROMOSOMES
We inherit chromosomes from our biological parents. Chromosomal abnormalities can cause disease or developmental problems.

SURROUNDINGS
If a child grows up deprived, it can impair development of areas related to memory, language processing, and decision-making.

GENES
Nearly every person has a full set of genes, but each gene may come in one of several varieties, and can determine our strengths and weaknesses.

BRAIN HEALTH

STRESS LEVELS
Chronic emotional stress in children can restrict the growth of neuron connections and lead to problems with memory, emotion, and learning.

GENE EXPRESSION
Genes produce chemicals that build the individual. This production work is known as gene expression. It can be sped up, slowed down, or even stopped.

GENETIC FACTORS

ENVIRONMENTAL FACTORS

DIET
A healthy diet rich in antioxidants, B vitamins, and Omega-3 fatty acids has been linked to maintaining brain functions in older people.

SOCIAL NETWORKS
Maintaining close social ties with friends and family can support memory and thinking skills and keep your brain stimulated.

IQ AND TWINS

Many research studies have looked at the connection between IQ—a measure of intelligence—and twins. Identical twins, who share the same genes, have been found in general to share a near identical IQ when they are brought up together, with little divergence in later life. Those who were raised separately were found to have only marginally different scores. In other words, environment has an effect, but so do genes.

At least one-third of all our genes are primarily active in the brain

RAISED TOGETHER OR APART
In one study, the difference in IQ of different siblings was measured. Identical twins had the highest similarity, whether they were raised together or not.

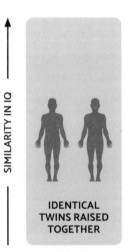
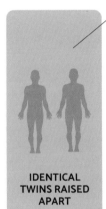
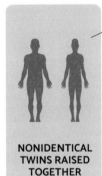
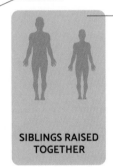
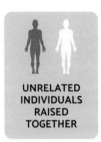

SIMILARITY IN IQ

Identical twins have the same genes, so differences in their IQ when they are raised apart must be due to environmental effects

Nonidentical twins are no more similar in their genes than any siblings; when raised together, their genetic differences lead to large IQ differences

Siblings are no more different in their genes than nonidentical twins, but they grew up at different times—variation in upbringing has made them more different in IQ

IDENTICAL TWINS RAISED TOGETHER

IDENTICAL TWINS RAISED APART

NONIDENTICAL TWINS RAISED TOGETHER

SIBLINGS RAISED TOGETHER

UNRELATED INDIVIDUALS RAISED TOGETHER

EPIGENETICS

[handwritten note]
Epigenetics
- Stress causes changes in person DNA
when person has offspring it inherits the altered DNA leads to depression and anxiety

...ing the ...es. Brain ...ir job, the ...mselves. If ...produces

hormones that can cause chemical changes in their DNA, and this can then prevent certain genes from being expressed. These changes in the DNA can then be inherited, meaning that the effect of the extreme stress can pass down to successive generations.

Stress hormones cause chemical changes in the person's DNA, although genetic code stays the same

The person's offspring may inherit this altered DNA and would be more likely to suffer depression and anxiety

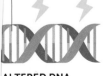

ALTERED DNA

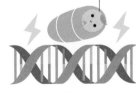

OFFSPRING

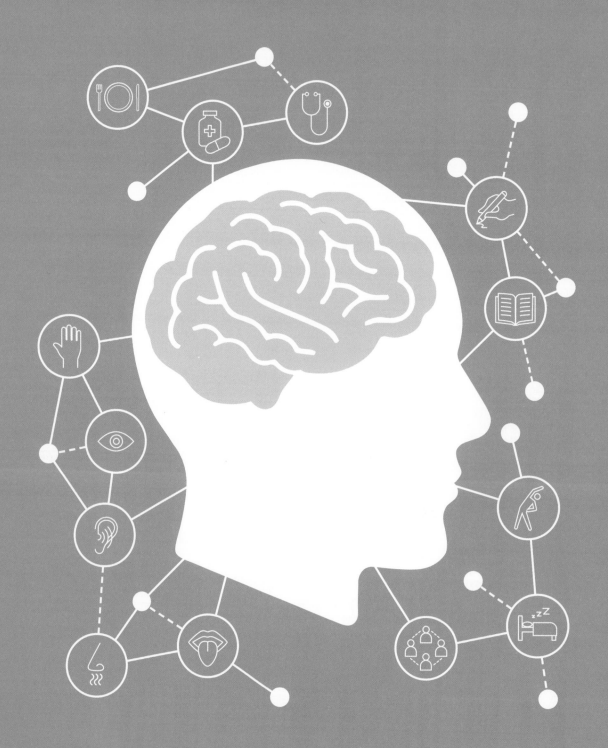

BRAIN
WORKOUT

GOOD BRAIN HEALTH

Like every other part of your body, your brain needs to be in good shape physically to work well. Exercise, rest, and good nutrition are therefore the building blocks of a bright mind.

BUSY BRAIN CELLS

In addition to being physically healthy, your brain needs to be mentally stimulated to function well. Activities that make you excited or cheerful have a direct effect on brain tissue by triggering electrical activity in your brain cells. Unused cells wither and may even die, whereas active cells produce growth chemicals and help to protect existing neural pathways and develop new ones.

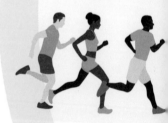

KEEP FIT
Exercise helps to keep your brain cells active, and to stave off anxiety or depression. One brisk walk each day is enough to make a difference.

EXERCISE
Regular exercise stimulates the brain as well as keeping the rest of your body fit–but you do not have to run a marathon to achieve this. Scans of electrical activity in the brain have revealed that a single 20-minute walk generates activity across the whole brain, even while resting afterward.

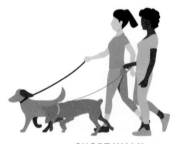

SHORT WALK

STAY SLIM

Obesity has long been linked to an increased risk of heart disease, cancer, and diabetes, but it is also bad for the brain. One study of more than 500 adults between ages 20 and 87 showed that obesity speeds up age-related brain shrinkage to the extent that the density of white matter (the pathways that carry information around the brain) in an overweight or obese person is equivalent to that of a slim person who is 10 years older. Obesity is defined as having a Body Mass Index (BMI) of 30 or more. A healthy BMI is between 18.5 and 25.

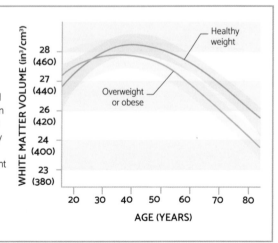

WHITE MATTER VOLUME (in³/cm³)

28 (460)
27 (440)
26 (420)
24 (400)
23 (380)

Healthy weight

Overweight or obese

20 30 40 50 60 70 80

AGE (YEARS)

GET PLENTY OF REST
While we sleep, our memories are consolidated and debris is washed out of the brain. Aim for 6–8 hours a night and avoid unscheduled naps, which may upset your body clock.

EAT WELL
Eating fresh food that is rich in vitamins and minerals (such as fruits and vegetables) helps to prevent strokes, which are one of the main causes of dementia.

SOCIALIZE
Interacting with other people, whether face-to-face or online, keeps you open to new experiences and helps you to avoid loneliness and depression.

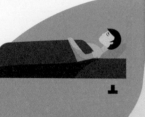
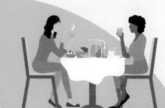
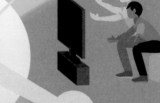
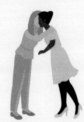
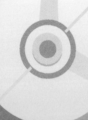
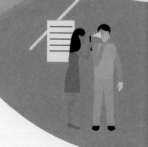
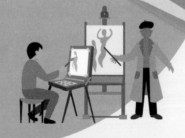

LOOK AFTER YOURSELF
Preserve your senses by having regular checkups, particularly for hearing and sight loss. Don't smoke or take recreational drugs or drink excessive amounts of alcohol.

STAY BUSY
Learning new things and staying intellectually active builds new brain tissue. Read lots of books, learn a new skill, and get a handle on the latest technology to keep your brain in gear.

THE REGIME
Generally, the brain thrives on the same things that keep your heart in good shape—a healthy diet, sleep, and exercise. Spending time with others and learning new things are also great for the brain.

ENEMIES OF THE BRAIN

The brain is a physical organ and needs to be looked after just like any other. Unlike other organs, it needs to be nurtured mentally, as well.

OBESITY

Hunger is controlled by a complex network including the brain, digestive system, and fat stores, but seeing food or feeling stressed can trigger a desire to eat whether or not you are hungry. Excess body fat can cause areas of the brain to swell or shrink, affecting hormone production and memory.

EXCESS ALCOHOL

Although the occasional glass of wine may be beneficial, long-term heavy drinking is very bad for the brain. It destroys brain cells and may even lead to a form of dementia called Korsakoff's psychosis.

THREATS TO PHYSICAL HEALTH

You can protect your brain by avoiding toxins such as tobacco and recreational drugs and limiting your alcohol intake. Maintaining a healthy weight through a balanced diet and regular exercise will also help to reduce or delay brain shrinkage and cognitive decline.

SMOKING

Smoking is a main cause of cardiovascular disease, which in turn increases the risk of stroke and dementia. Nicotine may help protect against Parkinson's disease, but the overall health hazards of smoking outweigh that possible benefit.

DRUGS

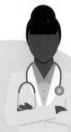

Taking recreational drugs can lead to life-wrecking addiction. Medicinal drugs may also cause cognitive problems as a side-effect—for example, drugs prescribed for anxiety may make you feel less alert. See your doctor if you suspect this.

Mental illnesses like depression are becoming more common

NEED FOR NOVELTY

Familiar thoughts and behavior stimulate the brain less and less over time. Trying new things (see pp.80–81), such as taking a cooking class or rethinking established beliefs, produces a rush of activity in the brain. If you constantly seek new experiences, you'll help maintain widespread brain activity.

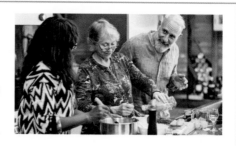

THREATS TO MENTAL HEALTH

Mental health is as important as physical health. Stress, trauma, pessimism, and loneliness can be managed through therapy or medication or, in less severe cases, by seeing friends or trying something new. Exercising your mind as well as your body should help to keep it healthy as you get older.

STRESS

Everyone suffers periods of stress, be they work-, money-, or health-related. Our bodies respond by producing cortisol (among other things), which helps in the short term but damages the brain in the long term.

NEGATIVITY

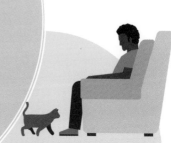

Negative thinking, and its extreme form, depression, is associated with the death of neurons. Drug treatments can reverse depression, but you may need to try a few to find one that works. Cognitive behavioral therapy can teach you how to be positive.

TRAUMA

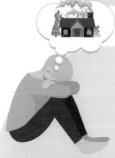

Terrifying or damaging events create memories that are difficult to erase because they are stored in the amygdala–an unconscious brain area that generates negative emotions. This can lead to post-traumatic stress disorder.

ISOLATION

Our brains have evolved specific circuitry that comes into play when we interact with other people. Like any other part of the brain, these connections need to be exercised to prevent them from wasting away.

REST AND SLEEP

Good sleep is essential for brain fitness. It helps to order our waking experiences, turn new ones into memories so they can be recalled, and protect the brain from physical decline.

One in five older people complain of restless legs. Exercise, baths, and stretching may help

SLEEP HYGIENE

Some people are lucky enough to fall asleep immediately, and to sleep for seven hours or more. Others find sleep difficult, especially as they get older. All sorts of things can cause insomnia or disturbed sleep, such as sleep apnea–when oxygen intake is reduced during sleep, or restless legs–an uncontrollable urge to move your legs that stops you from sleeping. Even so, it helps to establish what is known as "sleep hygiene"–a set of habits designed to result in a good night's sleep.

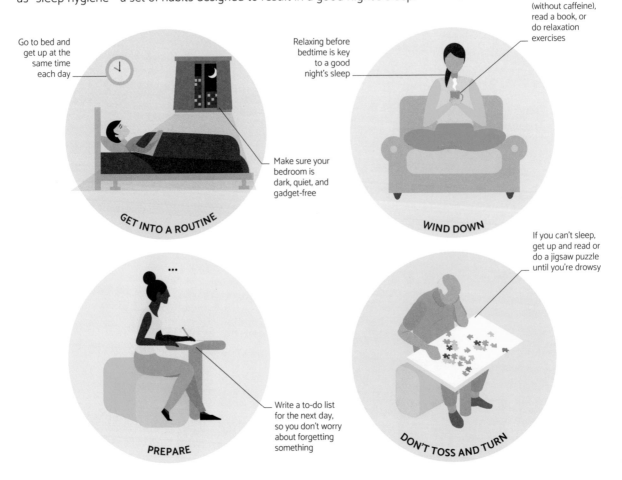

Go to bed and get up at the same time each day

Make sure your bedroom is dark, quiet, and gadget-free

GET INTO A ROUTINE

Relaxing before bedtime is key to a good night's sleep

Have a hot drink (without caffeine), read a book, or do relaxation exercises

WIND DOWN

Write a to-do list for the next day, so you don't worry about forgetting something

PREPARE

If you can't sleep, get up and read or do a jigsaw puzzle until you're drowsy

DON'T TOSS AND TURN

THE NEED FOR SLEEP

Tiny clumps of protein accumulate in the brain as a result of normal brain function. Sleep provides a quiet window for the brain to flush out this debris with cerebrospinal fluid before more can be formed. An abnormal buildup of protein clumps is associated with Alzheimer's disease, possibly because it restricts blood flow and obstructs neural signals.

Sleep is also vital for making memories. During deep sleep, the hippocampus (the part of the brain that encodes new information) sends neural signals to the cortex, carrying information about recent events. Once this transfer is complete, events are safely encoded in the cortex, where they remain as memories, provided the tissue is healthy.

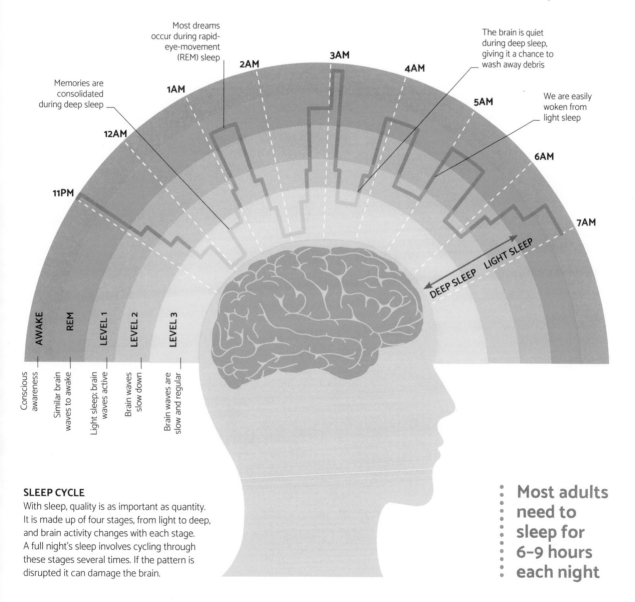

Most dreams occur during rapid-eye-movement (REM) sleep

The brain is quiet during deep sleep, giving it a chance to wash away debris

Memories are consolidated during deep sleep

We are easily woken from light sleep

2AM 3AM 4AM
1AM 5AM
12AM 6AM
11PM 7AM

AWAKE

REM

LEVEL 1

LEVEL 2

LEVEL 3

DEEP SLEEP   LIGHT SLEEP

Conscious awareness

Similar brain waves to awake

Light sleep; brain waves active

Brain waves slow down

Brain waves are slow and regular

SLEEP CYCLE
With sleep, quality is as important as quantity. It is made up of four stages, from light to deep, and brain activity changes with each stage. A full night's sleep involves cycling through these stages several times. If the pattern is disrupted it can damage the brain.

Most adults need to sleep for 6–9 hours each night

PHYSICAL ACTIVITY

Exercise is as important to the brain as it is to every other part of the body. It protects against cognitive decline and may even reduce the effects of dementia.

MENTAL WORKOUT

Regular exercise produces dramatic improvements in brain function. One study tracked physical activity levels and cognitive skills in a group of nearly 500 adults over 20 years. Those who exercised most scored better on memory and thinking tests and were significantly less likely to develop dementia. You don't need to run miles—exercising for an hour, three times a week, is enough to make a difference.

Being active doesn't have to mean running. Climbing stairs, swimming, or raking leaves all help keep your brain in good shape

GET FIT

If you struggle to get off the sofa, try joining an exercise class or making a regular arrangement to work out with a friend. Set yourself goals, such as walking a certain number of steps each day.

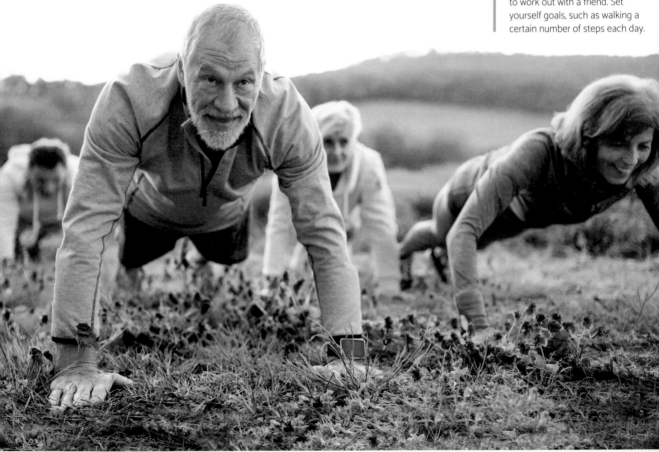

1 BRAIN FOOD
Moving around raises the heart rate, increasing the flow of oxygen- and nutrient-rich blood to the brain.

2 ACTIVATED CELLS
Increased levels of oxygen stimulate the neurons (brain cells), causing them to become more active.

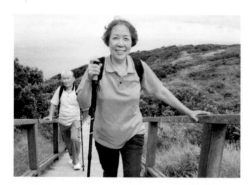

HAPPY HIKERS
All forms of exercise benefit the brain, but some have an exceptional effect on certain functions. Brisk walking, jogging, and dancing improve memory, thinking, and mood.

2. Neurons receive more oxygen, so become more active

3. BDNF helps neurons to stay healthy and grow new connections

1. Blood flow to the brain increases

4. "Feel-good" neurotransmitters are released

BRAIN IN ACTION

Physical activity has a marked effect on brain tissue, producing altered cognition by encouraging neurons to become active and to communicate with each other—the basis of all thinking. Since large parts of the brain are devoted to body movement, physical exercise automatically creates activity in large clusters of neurons. It also triggers the release of stress-busting chemicals, helping us to feel good.

3 CELL GROWTH
Exercise increases production of the protein brain-derived neurotrophic factor (BDNF), which helps neurons to form new connections and protects them from damage.

4 MOOD BOOST
Greater levels of neurotransmitters such as dopamine and endorphins are also released, boosting energy levels and mood and reducing stress.

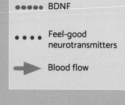

KEY

●●●●● BDNF

●●●● Feel-good neurotransmitters

➡ Blood flow

READING AND WRITING

We must all learn to read and write as children, but this is just the start of the story. The whole brain is required to maintain language skills, so reading and writing are vital to good brain health.

BROADENING THE MIND

Unlike talking and walking, reading and writing do not come naturally—they are too recent an acquisition for evolution to have written these abilities into our genes. Every individual has to be taught to read and write, and becoming literate is one of the most challenging things humans do because it involves creating new connections in the brain as well as putting old ones to a new use.

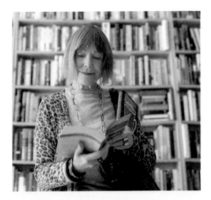

READING
In addition to being a relaxing and informative pastime, reading a good book improves your attention skills by focusing the mind on a single stimulus.

IMPROVING RECALL

Writing exercises parts of the brain concerned with structure and memory, while storytelling involves parts concerned with empathy and prediction, as well as memory. Keeping a written record of your daily experiences helps you to remember them because it forces you to bring them back to mind in order to describe them. The more often events are remembered, the more likely they are to stick.

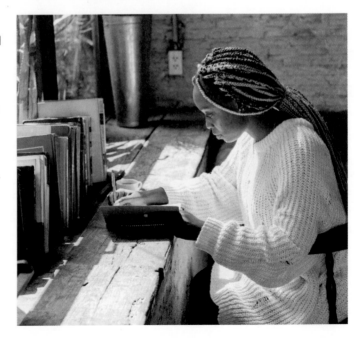

FINDING THE RIGHT WORDS
Extensive reading helps us to build up our vocabulary, while writing things down gives us the chance to use new words and therefore remember them.

USING THE WHOLE BRAIN

Reading and writing are among the best brain workouts you can do, because literacy exercises a wider range of brain areas than almost anything else. If you consider that in addition to these brain regions, areas are also activated by thinking about, or engaging emotionally with, the content of the literature, practically every part of the brain is exercised.

Reading people-based fiction has been found to improve a person's capacity for empathy

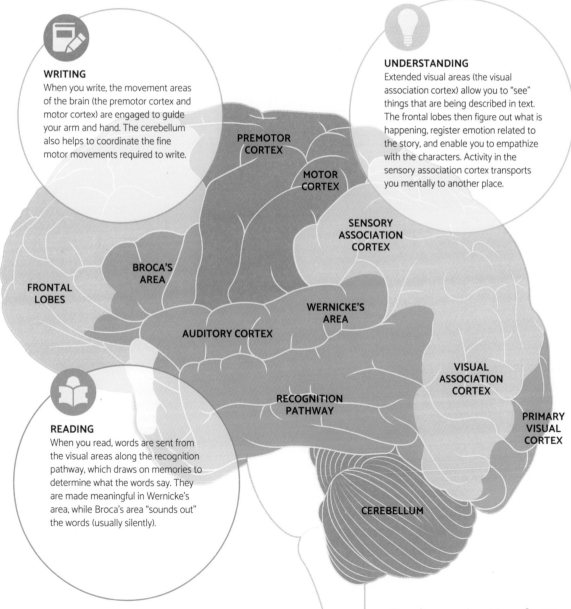

WRITING
When you write, the movement areas of the brain (the premotor cortex and motor cortex) are engaged to guide your arm and hand. The cerebellum also helps to coordinate the fine motor movements required to write.

UNDERSTANDING
Extended visual areas (the visual association cortex) allow you to "see" things that are being described in text. The frontal lobes then figure out what is happening, register emotion related to the story, and enable you to empathize with the characters. Activity in the sensory association cortex transports you mentally to another place.

READING
When you read, words are sent from the visual areas along the recognition pathway, which draws on memories to determine what the words say. They are made meaningful in Wernicke's area, while Broca's area "sounds out" the words (usually silently).

PREMOTOR CORTEX

MOTOR CORTEX

SENSORY ASSOCIATION CORTEX

BROCA'S AREA

FRONTAL LOBES

WERNICKE'S AREA

AUDITORY CORTEX

VISUAL ASSOCIATION CORTEX

RECOGNITION PATHWAY

PRIMARY VISUAL CORTEX

CEREBELLUM

DIGITAL TECHNOLOGY

Used appropriately, digital technology can help our brains stay sharp, make our lives more interesting, and enrich our interactions with other people.

Although socializing online is no substitute for face-to-face meetings, among older people, the use of social media is associated with a greater sense of well-being

COMPUTER LITERACY

Learning to use digital devices is becoming increasingly necessary as everyday activities like banking, shopping, and paying bills shift online. People who grew up using computers and mobile phones seem to have a natural ability to use them, while those who come to it later may struggle. One reason for this is that learning to use digital technology through play—as most young people do—establishes the activity as fun and links it to the pleasure areas of the brain. Those who learn as adults think "work" and link it with brain areas generating caution and fear.

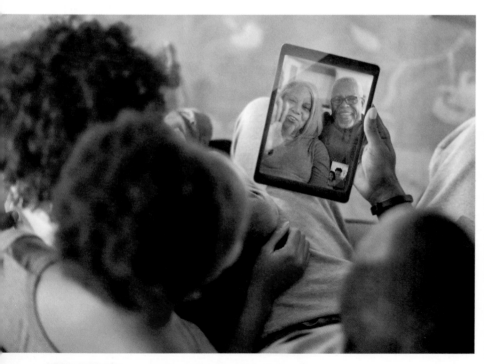

KEEP IN TOUCH
Rather than setting out to "learn how to use a tablet," start by finding something you want to do—such as talking to friends or family—and learn how to achieve that goal. Your digital skills will improve rapidly.

HELPFUL TECHNOLOGY

For those suffering from vision or hearing loss, voice recognition technology can help. Devices that use and understand human speech allow you to use computers and other digital devices, which might be difficult to manipulate by sight. You can instruct them to make phone or video calls, or type dictated messages. They can also produce subtitles to live conversations.

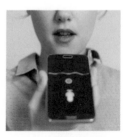

VOICE ASSISTANT

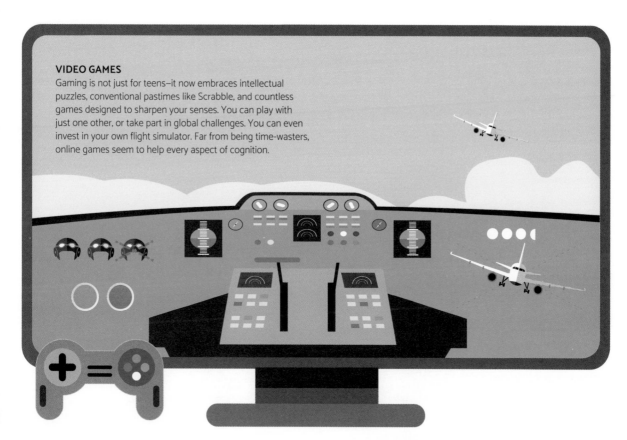

VIDEO GAMES

Gaming is not just for teens—it now embraces intellectual puzzles, conventional pastimes like Scrabble, and countless games designed to sharpen your senses. You can play with just one other, or take part in global challenges. You can even invest in your own flight simulator. Far from being time-wasters, online games seem to help every aspect of cognition.

EMBRACE TECHNOLOGY

At the start of the digital age, people panicked that computers would rob people of sustained attention and thinking abilities. While continuous gaming and destructive social interaction can cause problems, such as stress or anxiety, digital technology also offers a variety of cognitive challenges and positive social opportunities. Social media helps people to interact with others, relieving loneliness and sparking interest. Researchers have found that regular game-playing over time by adults improved their thinking, attention, emotional acuity, and spatial-reasoning skills.

BRAIN FITNESS GAMES

Unlike video games, brain games are marketed specifically to exercise your brain. The best ones are "suites," which include games designed for spatial learning, recognition, numbers, and words, along with rising levels of skill and built-in evaluation. However, it remains unclear whether the progress you make will translate into better cognition overall.

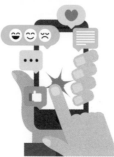

SOCIAL MEDIA

Used by young people to compare themselves with their peers, social media can lead to low self-esteem. But those who use it to keep in touch with friends and family are less likely to be depressed. Some studies have linked frequent social media use with better "executive function"—the sort of brain activity that organizes and plans.

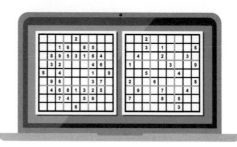

NUMBERS GAME

DIET AND THE BRAIN

The brain is a hungry organ, consuming about one-fifth of the body's calorie intake. Brain food is carried in blood, so a brain-healthy diet is one that keeps the delivery system flowing.

HEALTHY PLATEFUL
This plate shows what proportions of each food group you should be eating, although recommendations vary from country to country. Sugar, saturated fats, and highly processed foods should be avoided or eaten rarely. It is also important to drink plenty of water.

BALANCED DIET

A diet based on vegetables and whole grains, with moderate amounts of lean meat, fish, and dairy and limited quantities of fat, oil, sugar, and processed foods, should provide all the nutrients the brain needs to stay healthy. Supplementary vitamins and minerals are not normally necessary—however, older people may not absorb nutrients from food efficiently, and food may lose nutrients if stored. A daily multivitamin and mineral supplement may therefore be a useful addition.

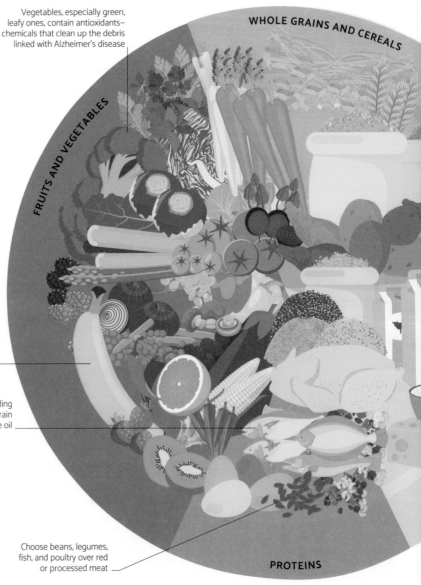

Vegetables, especially green, leafy ones, contain antioxidants—chemicals that clean up the debris linked with Alzheimer's disease

WHOLE GRAINS AND CEREALS

FRUITS AND VEGETABLES

Fruits and vegetables provide many of the vitamins and minerals needed to keep brain cells functioning

Fish is good for building and maintaining brain cells, as is olive oil

Choose beans, legumes, fish, and poultry over red or processed meat

PROTEINS

Eating a balanced, mostly plant-based diet and maintaining a healthy weight can help to delay cognitive decline

MINDFUL EATING

Researchers have devised three diets that are proven to protect against cognitive decline and dementia. They are similar in content, but vary in emphasis and in the extent to which they prescribe what you should eat and when–depending on whether your goal is to maintain a healthy weight or lose weight. All three diets recommend eating lots of green vegetables, olive oil, and whole grains, and moderate amounts of lean meat and fish.

Whole grains contain B vitamins, which are especially important for brain metabolism

DIET		FOOD
MEDITERRANEAN	The Mediterranean diet is based on the eating habits of people in that part of the world, who are exceptionally long-lived. Rich in vegetables, fruits, starchy foods, and olive oil, it appears to slow cognitive decline and protect against Alzheimer's disease.	• Whole grains, fruits and vegetables, olive oil, beans, nuts (every meal) • Fish and seafood (2+ servings/week) • Poultry, eggs, cheese, yogurt (3 servings of each/week) • Meat, pastry, sugar (1–2 servings/week) • Alcohol (1 small glass/day, preferably red wine)
DASH	Primarily designed to reduce blood pressure (a risk factor for dementia), the DASH (Dietary Approaches to Stop Hypertension) diet is also associated with good and improving cognition. It is based mostly on fruits and vegetables, along with whole grains and low-fat or fat-free dairy products.	• Whole grains (7–8 servings/day) • Vegetables (4–5 servings/day) • Fruits (4–5 servings/day) • Dairy: low-fat or fat-free (2–3 servings/day) • Lean meat, poultry, fish (no more than 2 servings/day) • Nuts, seeds, beans (4–5 servings/week) • Fats, oils (2–3 servings/day) • Sweets, desserts (no more than 5 servings/week)
MIND	The MIND (Mediterranean-DASH Intervention for Neurodegenerative Delay) diet is a combination of the Mediterranean and DASH diets, with emphasis on the elements known to be especially good for the brain. Butter and margarine, cheese, red meat, fried food, and sweets should be avoided or strictly limited.	• Green, leafy vegetables (6+ servings/week) • Berries (2+ servings/week) • Nuts (5+ servings/week) • Olive oil (use as main cooking oil) • Whole grains (3+ servings/day) • Fish, especially oily fish (1+ servings/week) • Beans (4+ servings/week) • Chicken or turkey (2+ servings/week, not fried) • Wine (maximum 1 glass/day)

DAIRY

OILS AND SPREADS

KETO DIET

Not suitable for those with preexisting health conditions, the keto diet involves cutting out carbohydrates, including pasta and fruit, and eating more proteins and fats, such as meat and dairy. Unlike other tissues, the brain can't use fatty acids as an energy source, so the liver converts them into ketone bodies for brain cells to use instead of carbohydrate-derived glucose. Used for a short time, the keto diet is good for weight loss, but it also seems to benefit the brain by reducing inflammation and inhibiting the oxidants that create the debris in the brain associated with dementia.

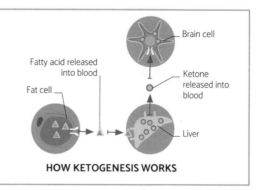

HOW KETOGENESIS WORKS

SUPPLEMENTS AND DRUGS

Thousands of substances are claimed to enhance cognition in healthy people, or improve it in those with failing skills, but the benefits–and risks–of taking them remain unclear.

WONDER ROOT?
Ginseng has been used in Chinese medicine for thousands of years, although scientific evidence of its benefits is limited.

NATURAL BRAIN BOOSTERS

Practically every product touted as "brain food" has failed to pass the stringent tests required to prove it works. This doesn't mean these products don't work–simply that scientific proof is missing. If you want to try a cognitive enhancer, first find out as much as you can about it. In particular, make sure it is safe when combined with any medications you are already taking, and never take more than the recommended dose. Even products labeled "natural" can cause side effects. Most natural substances claimed to help brain power are found in food, and a brain-healthy diet (see pp. 40–41) will deliver them all.

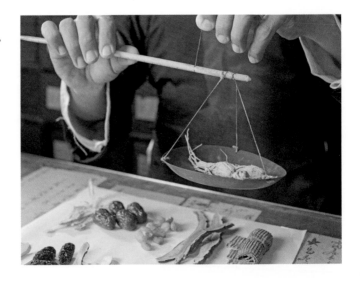

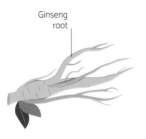

Ginseng root

GINSENG
One of the most popular herbal supplements available, ginseng is said to offer a fast-acting boost to learning and memory. It works by stimulating a neurotransmitter called acetylcholine. Scientific evidence remains weak, however.

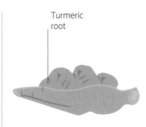

Turmeric root

CURCUMIN
Curcumin is derived from the turmeric root. There is evidence to suggest that it enhances memory and promotes the growth of new neurons by raising levels of a natural brain protein that stimulates cell growth.

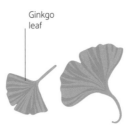

Ginkgo leaf

GINKGO BILOBA
Millions swear by ginkgo biloba, which is said to be good for memory, attention, and anxiety. Claims that it improves blood flow to the brain and cleans up detritus, protecting against dementia, remain to be proven scientifically.

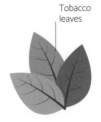

Tobacco leaves

NICOTINE
Although smoking tobacco is extremely harmful, nicotine on its own has been scientifically shown to help concentration, memory, and imagination. It also seems to guard against Parkinson's disease and possibly prevent Alzheimer's.

MEDICINAL DRUGS

Several prescription drugs that were developed for certain conditions have been found to have cognitive enhancing effects. Like all drugs, they can also have severe side effects, and can interact harmfully with other medication. They should not be taken without a prescription, nor for any reason other than that for which they were prescribed. The unlicensed use of "smart drugs" by healthy people could be dangerous.

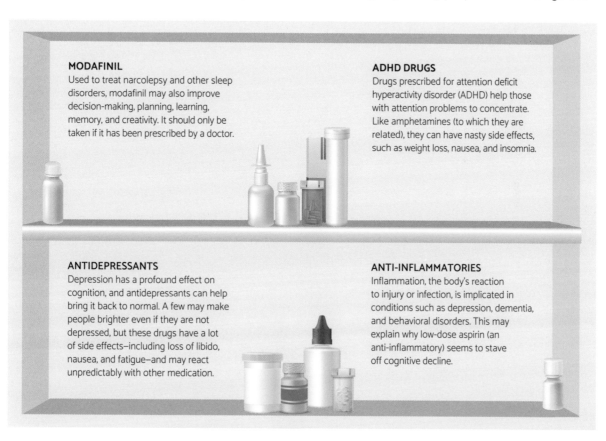

MODAFINIL
Used to treat narcolepsy and other sleep disorders, modafinil may also improve decision-making, planning, learning, memory, and creativity. It should only be taken if it has been prescribed by a doctor.

ADHD DRUGS
Drugs prescribed for attention deficit hyperactivity disorder (ADHD) help those with attention problems to concentrate. Like amphetamines (to which they are related), they can have nasty side effects, such as weight loss, nausea, and insomnia.

ANTIDEPRESSANTS
Depression has a profound effect on cognition, and antidepressants can help bring it back to normal. A few may make people brighter even if they are not depressed, but these drugs have a lot of side effects–including loss of libido, nausea, and fatigue–and may react unpredictably with other medication.

ANTI-INFLAMMATORIES
Inflammation, the body's reaction to injury or infection, is implicated in conditions such as depression, dementia, and behavioral disorders. This may explain why low-dose aspirin (an anti-inflammatory) seems to stave off cognitive decline.

> Many "smart drugs" can have nasty or even harmful side effects, and most are not tested beyond their intended use

TRANSCRANIAL DIRECT CURRENT STIMULATION
The brain runs on electricity, and sending a tiny current through the skull can enhance its natural activity. Transcranial direct current stimulation (tDCS) is a safe, painless treatment that delivers the charge through electrodes. Possible benefits include reducing anxiety, stimulating memory and attention, and alleviating headaches–although the degree of effect is still questionable.

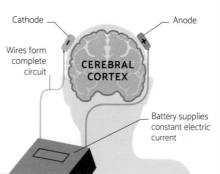

Cathode

Anode

Wires form complete circuit

CEREBRAL CORTEX

Battery supplies constant electric current

KEEPING YOUR SENSES

As we age, our senses tend to become less sharp. To keep your brain function up to speed, make sure your eyesight, hearing, and other senses are as good as they can be.

About half of all people in Europe wear glasses, and nearly everyone over the age of 75 needs them for close work

PROPRIOCEPTION
The brain processes signals from joints, tendons, and muscles, allowing us to sense our body without looking.

TASTE
Taste works alongside smell to give us enjoyment from food and to determine what is safe to eat.

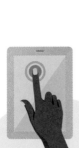

TOUCH
Touch allows us to make physical contact with the world. Nerves under the skin register stimulation, including pain.

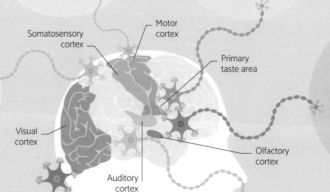

Somatosensory cortex

Motor cortex

Primary taste area

Visual cortex

Olfactory cortex

Auditory cortex

SMELL
Smell goes straight to the emotional brain area, giving us joy. It also detects danger, such as from gas or smoke.

SIGHT
Sight is most people's main way of knowing the world, and failing sight is linked to cognitive decline.

THE WORLD AROUND US

Our eyes, ears, nose, tongue, and peripheral nerves constantly feed our brains with information from the environment. The brain turns this into sights, sounds, tastes and smells, and awareness of our bodies. If the information flow is reduced, the brain cells that usually process it become less active, and so the sensations become less vivid.

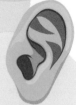

SOUND
Human communication often relies on hearing, so losing this sense easily creates social isolation.

FAILING SENSES

Our senses tend to fail gradually and it is easy not to notice sensory impairment until it starts to impinge on daily living. A person may realize they are stumbling, ignoring the newspaper because it is an effort to read, or zoning out of conversations because they are too difficult to follow. Other drivers may hoot at them for reasons they don't understand. By this point, the brain may already be slightly damaged, so it is important to monitor your senses regularly to make sure that impairment is noticed and corrected immediately.

		PROBLEM	ACTION	REMEDY
SOUND		Do you find conversations or TV programs hard to follow? Do you struggle to hear in a crowd?	Get your hearing tested. If you suspect you have hidden hearing problems not identified by a basic test, ask for more tests.	Hearing aid.
SIGHT		Do you struggle to read or recognize objects or people? Are images indistinct, and do you find yourself being clumsy?	Get your eyes tested (see pp.46–47).	Glasses, cataract surgery, laser treatment.
TASTE		Does food seem bland? Have your cooking skills worsened?	See your doctor (for example, to check for a virus or infection, sinusitis, or dental problems).	Medical treatment (such as antibiotics for an infection), better mouth hygiene, taste exercises (see pp.46–47).
SMELL		Do you fail to notice the smell of burning, garbage, or rotten food?	Test your sense of smell (see pp.46–47) and see your doctor if you are concerned.	Medical treatment if required (such as nasal spray for sinusitis), smelling exercises at home.
BALANCE		Do you find yourself stumbling or swaying or becoming less coordinated than usual?	Test your proprioception (see pp.46–47) and go to your doctor if necessary.	Medical treatment (for example, for head injury or infection), exercises to improve peripheral-body-to-brain communication.

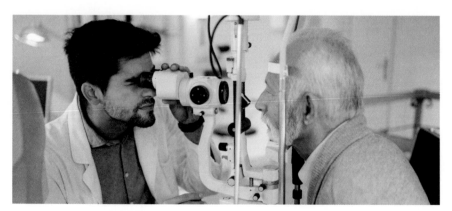

EYE TEST

Cataracts are common in older people, causing clouded vision and blindness if left untreated. If your vision is blurred, lights feel dazzling, or colors look faded, go to your optician. They will examine your eyes and test your vision and refer you for further treatment if required.

TESTING YOUR SENSES

Don't take your senses for granted. They are your doorway to the outside world, so check them regularly yourself to make sure they are working properly.

Worrying about the risk of falling makes you more likely to fall

EXERCISE 1 | TEST YOUR EYESIGHT

As you get older, you're more likely to have problems with your eyesight. The first sign is usually difficulty reading—you may need to hold a book farther away or use a brighter light to see details. You can buy reading glasses at pharmacies or online, but it's vital all the same to get your eyes checked by a specialist at least once every two years. Many sight problems can be treated best if caught early, and others may be secondary to an underlying illness such as diabetes.

ON THE SPOT
One common condition you can test for is macular degeneration, which affects the central field of vision. Focus on the spot in the middle of this grid. If the lines around it look wavy, see your doctor immediately. Rapid treatment can stop the condition from worsening.

EXERCISE 2 | TEST YOUR SENSE OF TOUCH

Sensitivity to touch, including pressure, temperature, and pain, changes with age. It may diminish due to reduced blood flow to the touch sensors in the skin, or because the sensors themselves, or the brain areas that read their signals, have become less responsive. Conversely, you may get more sensitive because of thinning skin. If you suspect you are becoming less sensitive, try monitoring the temperature of your bathwater. It is important to be aware of any changes to ensure that loss of touch does not put you in danger.

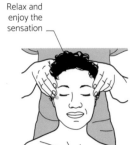

Relax and enjoy the sensation

① Gentle touch, such as in the form of a head massage, releases brain chemicals, which are good for your body and generate pleasure as well.

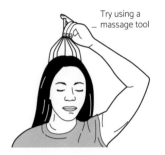

Try using a massage tool

② You can achieve the same soothing effect at home on your own—a light stroking movement at a speed of about 1 in (3 cm) a second is ideal.

EXERCISE 3 | TEST YOUR SMELL AND TASTE SENSES

Unlike other senses, smell directly excites the emotional part of the brain, creating meaning and pleasure. Taste works with it, enabling us to enjoy food. Both senses help us detect danger, such as from bad food or smoke, but they weaken with age as taste buds, and the nerves in the nose that register odors, shrink. Simple exercises can increase the size of your olfactory bulb (the part of the brain that registers smell).

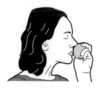

LEMON

ROSE   **MINT**   **CINNAMON**

(1) You can amplify your senses of smell and taste by concentrating on different scents and flavors. Choose four items you like to smell, and smell each for one minute.

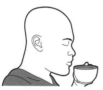

COFFEE

ROSEMARY **STAR ANISE** **BANANA**

(2) The next day, choose another four items and smell them. Gradually build up your "library" of different smells and check regularly that you can identify them.

EXERCISE 4 | TEST YOUR PROPRIOCEPTION

Proprioception (the sixth sense) tells us what is happening to our body—where it is in space and what it is doing. Like all our senses, it tends to get less efficient with age, making it more likely that we will fall over and hurt ourselves. Proprioception is largely unconscious—you use it every time you move—but it is possible to improve it consciously by deliberately unbalancing your body. This forces the proprioceptive pathways in your brain to work harder, and the harder they work, the better they get.

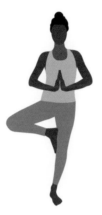

BALANCING ACT
Test your proprioception by standing on one leg. If you get wobbly after a few seconds, practice doing it for a little longer each day.

(1) It is hard to find your fingers with your eyes shut. Hold your left hand up with the fingers apart. Now touch your nose with your right index finger.

(2) Close your eyes. Move your right index finger to touch your left thumb. Then bring your right finger back to your nose.

(3) Try touching each finger on your left hand, bringing your right index finger back to your nose every time. Can you find your fingers each time?

ALONE IN A CROWD

Hidden hearing loss does not show up on the usual auditory test because it does not reduce a person's ability to hear quiet sounds. Rather, it makes it difficult to distinguish foreground sound from background noise. If you don't like trying to talk in a noisy room, or you often mishear a word, you might have the condition. This is most likely if you have been exposed to loud noise. Some new hearing aids can improve hidden hearing loss, so if you feel you have a problem even after having a "good" auditory test, press for more information.

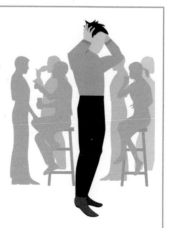

SOCIAL CONNECTIONS

The human brain has evolved for social living and needs the stimulation of others. People who are deprived of company show greater cognitive decline in later years than those who are social.

BETTER TOGETHER

Having close friends and a healthy social network is good for the brain. It is also likely that when individuals keep an active interest in new things it makes them more likely to seek out similar people to talk to, and their company in turn helps keep the individuals' brains alert, interested, and stimulated.

Having friends with similar interests encourages people to experience new things, which stimulates the brain

SUPER-AGERS

FRIENDS ARE . . .

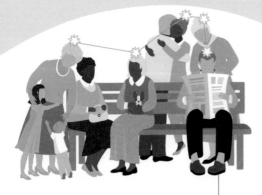

THE SUPER SECRET
A small number of people are dubbed "super-agers" because their brains seem to defy the aging process–they remain as sharp at 80 as most people are in middle-age. Studies have found that super-agers often report having extremely high levels of satisfaction in their social relationships. It could be that their high-quality social lives have enhanced their brains.

Super-agers are found to have more close friends than other people of the same age

SOCIAL STIMULATION
If a person has no one to accompany them, they are less likely to travel and try new things, which could deprive them of the sort of stimulation that keeps the brain active. Loneliness may also make people less inclined to look after themselves–for example, having a poor diet–which in turn may result in physical changes that impact on the brain.

Individuals who report feelings of loneliness are more likely to have health problems later in their life

Humans have evolved as a social species, which means that people unconsciously feel unsafe without the protection of "the herd"

...GOOD FOR THE BRAIN

BEING **ALONE**

LONELY BRAIN

It is possible to be lonely in a crowd–loneliness and social isolation are not the same thing. Both of them, though, seem to be bad for the brain, probably because in both states, people tend to have reduced mental stimulation. However, it may be possible to offset the many risks of being alone by keeping the brain active.

PHYSICAL BRAIN CHANGES

Loneliness or isolation can cause physical changes in the brain, which may then have knock-on effects on the rest of the body. Studies have indicated a number of different brain changes, including reduced volume in specific regions of the brain and higher stress hormone levels. When occurring over a long period, high levels of stress hormones have been shown to damage the brain.

Reduced brain volumes in the prefrontal cortex, a region important in decision-making and social behavior

Smaller-than-normal hippocampus, which is associated with impaired learning and memory

Amygdala, the part of the brain that generates emotions, is smaller in people who are lonely

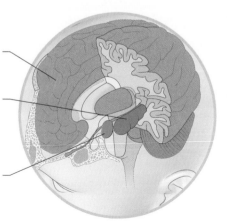

BRAIN OF A LONELY PERSON

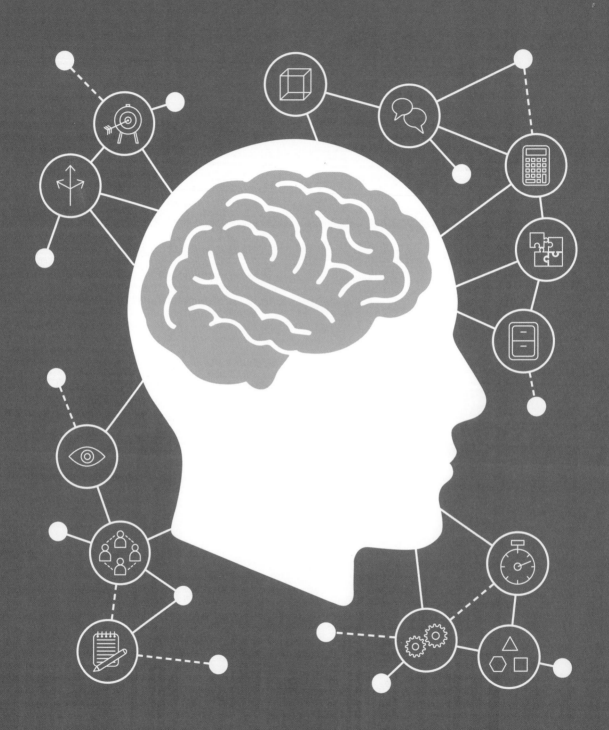

THINKING
SKILLS

MENTAL PROCESSES

Thinking is just one of the mental processes that are together known as cognition. Cognition is an umbrella term for the brain activity that produces all experience and behavior, both conscious and unconscious.

Multitasking is a myth—our brains are just constantly switching attention between tasks

CRYSTALLIZED OR FLUID

Some mental tasks involve retrieving information that you have already learned. Such tasks are called "crystallized." Tasks that involve processing new information are known as "fluid" cognition. Some mental tasks may involve both. Older people usually retain crystallized intelligence, but fluid cognition tends to decline with age.

SPECTRUM OF COGNITION
The spectrum of mental tasks, from crystallized to fluid, can also be roughly grouped into memory tasks, skills, and executive functions.

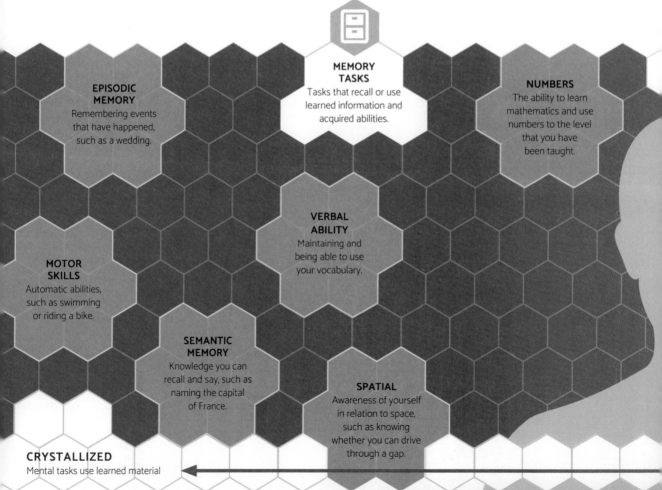

MEMORY TASKS
Tasks that recall or use learned information and acquired abilities.

EPISODIC MEMORY
Remembering events that have happened, such as a wedding.

NUMBERS
The ability to learn mathematics and use numbers to the level that you have been taught.

VERBAL ABILITY
Maintaining and being able to use your vocabulary.

MOTOR SKILLS
Automatic abilities, such as swimming or riding a bike.

SEMANTIC MEMORY
Knowledge you can recall and say, such as naming the capital of France.

SPATIAL
Awareness of yourself in relation to space, such as knowing whether you can drive through a gap.

CRYSTALLIZED
Mental tasks use learned material

EXPECTED DECLINE

Older people are more optimistic than those who are younger when it comes to predicting age-related cognitive decline. A survey of more than 3,000 individuals over the age of 40 found that the younger volunteers thought decline would set in a full 15 years earlier than those over age 70. All age groups assumed that their wisdom and knowledge would not decline until a much later age compared to their memory. Out of all the volunteers, 91 percent believed that there are things people can do to maintain or improve their cognitive skills.

CHANGING EXPECTATIONS

These bar charts show the age at which people in different age groups thought their cognitive skills would start to decline. All age groups assumed that their ability to remember things would be the first to decline.

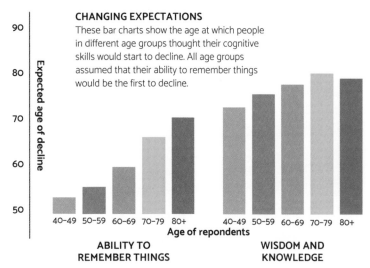

Expected age of decline

| 90 | 80 | 70 | 60 | 50 |

Age of repondents

40–49 50–59 60–69 70–79 80+

ABILITY TO REMEMBER THINGS

40–49 50–59 60–69 70–79 80+

WISDOM AND KNOWLEDGE

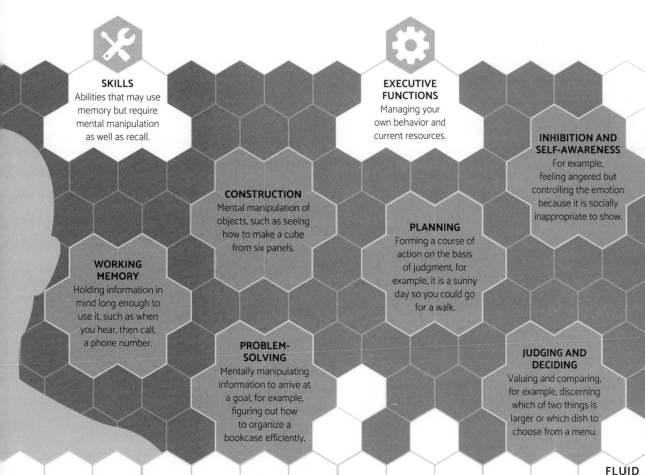

SKILLS
Abilities that may use memory but require mental manipulation as well as recall.

EXECUTIVE FUNCTIONS
Managing your own behavior and current resources.

INHIBITION AND SELF-AWARENESS
For example, feeling angered but controlling the emotion because it is socially inappropriate to show.

CONSTRUCTION
Mental manipulation of objects, such as seeing how to make a cube from six panels.

PLANNING
Forming a course of action on the basis of judgment, for example, it is a sunny day so you could go for a walk.

WORKING MEMORY
Holding information in mind long enough to use it, such as when you hear, then call, a phone number.

PROBLEM-SOLVING
Mentally manipulating information to arrive at a goal, for example, figuring out how to organize a bookcase efficiently.

JUDGING AND DECIDING
Valuing and comparing, for example, discerning which of two things is larger or which dish to choose from a menu.

FLUID
Mental tasks involve juggling new information

AM I NORMAL?

It's normal for mental abilities to decline with age, but when does normal age-related cognitive decline become something to worry about?

Short naps are healthy for the brain, as they allow areas of the brain to recover

COGNITIVE DECLINE

Age changes the way our brains work, not necessarily because the organ is "wearing out" or diseased but because we are genetically programmed to work differently at different ages. For example, older people may take longer to make a decision because they take more factors into account first. The most obvious changes, however, are due to simple age-related degeneration, just as wrinkles appear on our skin. Most aspects of cognition stay steady until middle age and then decline at slightly different rates.

WHAT IS NORMAL?

What is normal for one person is not normal for another. Each individual varies in their mental ability, not just across time but also according to whether, for example, they are stressed or ill. Some symptoms (see the next page for examples) may be a sign of "unhealthy" changes in your brain. If you are worried about your mental performance, visit your doctor.

DECLINING SKILLS

Cognitive abilities change at different rates. This graph represents one study in which people of different ages were tested at the same time and shows that some skills are maintained well into old age. Results differ slightly if only one group of people is tested as they age, with thinking speed declining first.

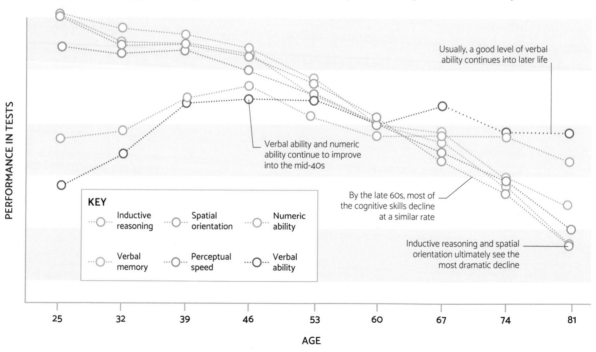

Usually, a good level of verbal ability continues into later life

Verbal ability and numeric ability continue to improve into the mid-40s

By the late 60s, most of the cognitive skills decline at a similar rate

Inductive reasoning and spatial orientation ultimately see the most dramatic decline

PERFORMANCE IN TESTS

KEY

- Inductive reasoning
- Spatial orientation
- Numeric ability
- Verbal memory
- Perceptual speed
- Verbal ability

AGE

25 32 39 46 53 60 67 74 81

		NORMAL SYMPTOMS	ABNORMAL SYMPTOMS
MEMORY		• Losing your keys occasionally • Entering a room and forgetting what you went there for • Failing to recognize an acquaintance	• Forgetting where you usually keep your keys • Finding yourself somewhere and not knowing how you got there • Failing to recognize close friends or family
ABILITY WITH WORDS		• Forgetting rarely used words • Occasionally getting words in the wrong order • Sometimes struggling to understand fast or unfamiliar dialogue	• Frequently forgetting common words • Unable to construct a sentence • Inability to get words "out" despite knowing them • Unable to follow a simple story
ABILITY WITH NUMBERS		• Needing to write down numbers in order to add them up • Having to check money or change a couple of times to ensure it's right • Difficulty counting backward	• Unable to say which of two numbers is greater • Unable to add, divide, or subtract with pen and paper • Unable to recall a four-digit PIN that you use every day
PROBLEM SOLVING		• Sometimes having difficulty seeing what a problem is—for example, taking a moment to realize the car will not start because it has run out of gas	• Failing to recognize a simple problem • Unable to think of how to begin finding a solution • Panicking when confronted with minor problems—for example, if pasta boils over on the stove
DECISION-MAKING		• Being occasionally indecisive • Dithering over what to choose from a menu	• Never being able to make a decision • Unable to complete purchases when shopping because of an inability to choose
ATTENTION AND FOCUS		• Forgetting what you are meant to be doing in the middle of a task • Boiling water in a kettle and forgetting to pour it into the teapot	• Unable to complete essential tasks without distraction • Unable to get dressed without distraction • Unable to make a cup of tea without distraction
THINKING AND REACTION TIME		• Being slow on the uptake • Noticing you have knocked a glass over, but being too slow to stop it from breaking	• Unable to cross a road because it feels like traffic is going too fast • Unable to catch a ball when thrown gently and accurately at you
SPATIAL VISUALIZATION		• Occasionally missing a step on the stairs • Bumping into a table • Not packing your shopping bags as efficiently as usual	• Unable to understand how a simple item of self-assembly furniture fits together • Unable to wrap a package in a minimum amount of paper

ABILITY TO RECALL

Memory is used in everything you do, and it is a key part of who you are. Practice consciously using it with the tests on these four pages. Note how difficult you found each one, to score yourself at the end.

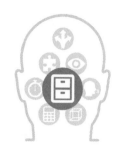

① SMILEY CIRCLES
Start by drawing five empty circles on a piece of paper, as shown below right, then spend 30 seconds studying the "smiley" faces on the left. When time is up, cover the faces and redraw them as accurately as you can within the five empty circles you drew.

② DIGITAL CHALLENGE
Using any technique you like, spend up to 30 seconds memorizing the row of 12 digits on the calculator display. When time is up, cover them up and write them out in order as accurately as you can.

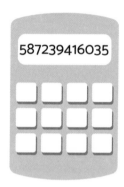

587239416035

③ OUT OF THIS WORLD
Start by covering the list of distances beneath the gray line, then read on. The list above the line gives the names of the eight largest moons of Jupiter, along with their approximate diameter in miles. Spend as long as you feel you need memorizing the list, then cover it up and see if you can recall which moon has each of the given diameters.

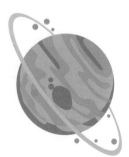

Ganymede	3,270
Callisto	2,995
Io	2,261
Europa	1,939
Amalthea	104
Himalia	87
Thebe	61
Elara	50

Which moon has each of the following diameters?

1,939 miles	87 miles
61 miles	104 miles
3,270 miles	

④ RESHAPED
Start by covering the second (lower) grid of shapes, then spend up to 1 minute studying the first (upper) grid. When time is up, cover the first grid and reveal the second. How many shapes have changed in appearance? Which ones?

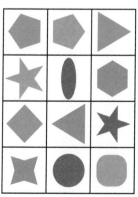

5 FACIAL RECALL

Spend as long as you feel is necessary memorizing the name associated with each of the following six faces. When you are ready, cover up the six named faces, leaving just the six unnamed copies of these faces. Can you recall the correct name for each of the faces?

DOUGLAS   MEENA   AHMED

SARAH   JAMES   YING

6 OBJECT LOCATION

Start by covering the question list below, then take a look at the following floorplan and the location of each of the objects shown. When time is up, cover up the floor plan and reveal the questions instead. How many of them can you answer? Keep track of your responses on a piece of paper, then check back to see how you did once you have answered them all.

1. In what room was the passport located?

2. Which two items were in the dining room?

3. What item, other than the umbrella, was in the study?

4. How many different items were marked on the map?

5. Which item was positioned farthest to the right on the map?

6. If you were to enter via the porch, which item would take longest to walk to?

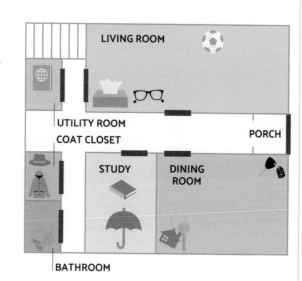

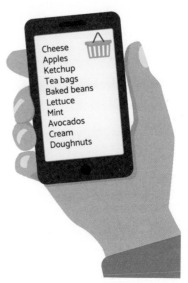

7 GROCERY LIST

Spend up to 2 minutes memorizing the grocery list above. Then, when time is up, cover it up and see how many of the 10 items you can recall.

8 VEGETABLE ACRONYMS

Spend just 1 minute studying the following three lists of vegetables, then cover them up and see how many you can recall. The first letters of each word in each set spell out a five-letter word. You can leave these words uncovered at the bottom as a reminder.

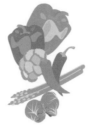

CARROT	**T**URNIP	**S**QUASH
OKRA	**R**ADISH	**M**USHROOM
ASPARAGUS	**A**RUGULA	**O**NION
CABBAGE	**I**CEBERG	**K**ALE
HORSERADISH	**L**ENTIL	**Y**AM
COACH	**TRAIL**	**SMOKY**

9 PASSWORD PROBLEMS

Remembering passwords and PINs can be a problem. Spend as long as you need to memorize the following list, then cover them up and see how well you can recall them when given the prompts.

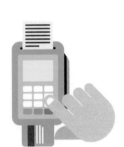

Bank password: **L3Tm3In**
ATM PIN: **1712**
Door code: ....**#31795***
Website login: ....**d0g5ar3gr8!**

Can you now recall each of these?:

Website login ....
Bank password ....
Door code ....
ATM PIN ....

10 RECIPE QUANTITIES

Cover up the partial ingredients list at the bottom of the clipboard, then study the full list at the top for no more than 1 minute. When time is up, cover the top and reveal the partial list beneath. Can you recall the missing items and quantities? Make a note of your answers on a piece of paper and then see how you did.

QUANTITY	ITEM
5	Eggs
3 cups	Flour
2 cups	Milk
2 tbsp	Sugar
1 tsp	Yeast
8 oz	Raisins

QUANTITY	ITEM
2 tbsp	——————
——————	Milk
8 oz	——————
——————	Eggs
——————	Yeast
3 cups	——————

11 EXTRA OBJECTS

Start by covering up the bottom set of objects below. Then, spend no more than 2 minutes studying the top arrangement of objects. When time is up, cover them up and reveal the bottom set. How many of these objects are new? Can you identify which ones?

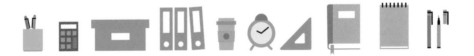

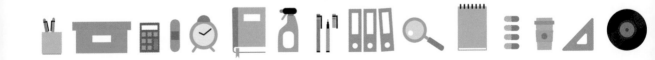

12 SOUTH AMERICA

When trying memory tests, it can be useful to memorize real-world information. If you are not already able to recall fully these countries and territories in South America, then spend as long as you need learning them. Then, when you are ready, cover up the labeled map and see if you can recall the names of all 13 countries and territories, using the blank map as a prompt.

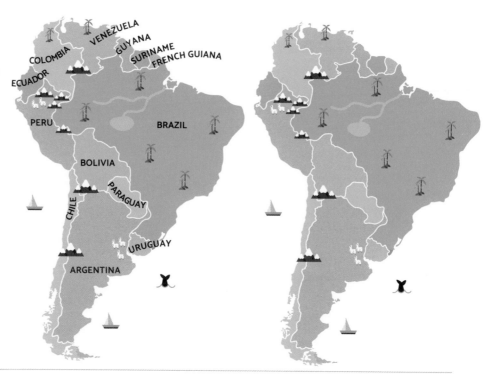

13 GRID MEMORY

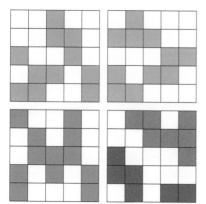

Start by drawing four 5x5 grids on a piece of paper. Then, for each of the patterns above, in turn, first look at it for no more than about 5 seconds. When 5 seconds is up, cover it up and see how accurately you can reproduce it on one of your grids by shading in the corresponding squares.

14 PLAYING CARDS

When playing cards, it can be useful to keep track of which cards have already been discarded. Study the following arrangement of cards for as long as you feel you need, then cover them up and see how many of the 12 cards you can recall.

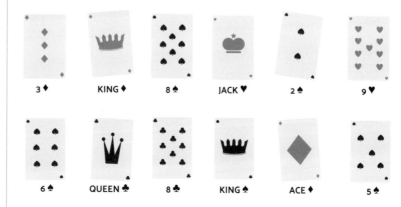

| 3 ♦ | KING ♦ | 8 ♠ | JACK ♥ | 2 ♠ | 9 ♥ |
| 6 ♠ | QUEEN ♣ | 8 ♣ | KING ♠ | ACE ♦ | 5 ♠ |

> **How did you find these tasks?** Rate the difficulty of each from 1 (hardest) to 3 (easiest) and add up your score.
>
> **14–22**: Your memory needs work. In chapter 4, try all the memory techniques and activities.
>
> **23–32**: Your memory is average. Use the techniques and activities with the memory icon in chapter 4 to boost your performance.
>
> **33–42**: Your memory is impressive, but to maintain it that way, keep practicing.

ABILITY WITH WORDS

The ability to communicate clearly is a key skill, and having a good vocabulary is a core part of that. Test your language abilities with the puzzles on these two pages.

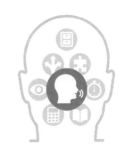

① ZIGZAG

Write a letter in each shaded square in order to form seven words. The last two letters of each word become the first two letters of the following word, in the same order, as indicated by the shaded connections.

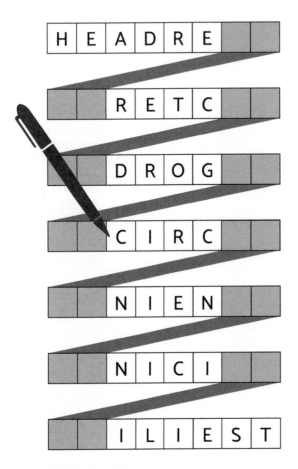

H	E	A	D	R	E		
		R	E	T	C		
	D	R	O	G			
		C	I	R	C		
	N	I	E	N			
	N	I	C	I			
	I	L	I	E	S	T	

✦ Answers on p.180

② WORD CHAINS

Complete each of these two word chains by writing a regular English word at each step. Every word must use the same letters in the same order as the word above it, but with a single letter changed. For example, you might change JOIN to LOIN, then to LOON, and so on.

✦ Answers on p.180

JOIN

QUIT

FIRM

SOON

③ SHIFTED LETTERS

All of the following words have had the same encoding applied, where each letter has been shifted by a fixed number of places through the alphabet. For example, A might have become B, B might have become C, and so on until Z became A. Can you crack the encoding and reveal the names of five birds?

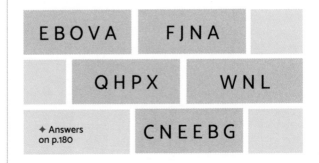

EBOVA

FJNA

QHPX

WNL

CNEEBG

✦ Answers on p.180

that visits
must spell
. The path
en squares.

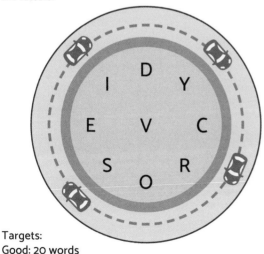

R D L B A I O F
A R O B E C B U
W R R P M U P T
R O I M A L N O

✦ Answer on p.180

✦ Answers
on p.180

⑤ LETTER SOUP

Can you rearrange these letters to reveal five colors? Each letter will be used exactly once, with no letters left over.

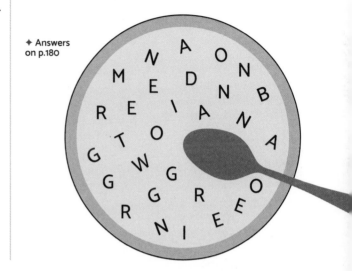

⑥ WORD CIRCLE

How many words can you form from this word circle? Every word must use the central letter plus two or more of the other letters, and no letter may be used more than once within any word. One word uses all of the letters.

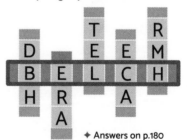

Targets:
Good: 20 words
Excellent: 30 words
Superb: 40 words

✦ Answers on p.180

⑦ FIVE FOR FIVE

Can you spell five different five-letter words using this word slider? To spell a word, imagine sliding each of the tabs up and down to reveal different letters through the central window. One word is spelled already to get you started.

Once you've found five words, for a much harder challenge, see if you can find four more words.

	T		R
D	E	E	M
B	**E**	**L**	**C**	**H**
H	R		A
	A		

✦ Answers on p.180

How many puzzles did you complete correctly?

0–3: Your verbal ability would benefit from substantial practice. In chapter 4, focus on activities with the "verbal skills" speech icon.

4–5: You have good basic ability with words, but could use more practice. Find chapter 4 word activities to boost your verbal skills..

6–7: Your ability with words is excellent. If you enjoy word challenges, stretch yourself further with the speech-icon activities in chapter 4.

ABILITY WITH NUMBERS

Being comfortable with handling numbers is important not just for managing your money but also for being able to think logically about many of life's challenges. Try these math exercises.

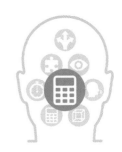

① NUMBER DARTS

Form each of the given totals by choosing one number from each ring of the dartboard, so that those three numbers add up to the desired total. For example, you could form a total of 55 by picking 15 from the center ring, 8 from the middle ring, and 32 from the outer ring.

TOTALS

60
70
85

✦ Answers on p.180

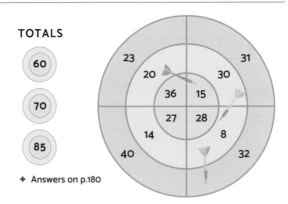

② CIRCLE NUMBERS

Can you figure out how to place a number from 1 to 9 into each circle, so no number is used more than once and so that each marked line adds up to the given total? You may find it handy to keep track of your deductions on a piece of scrap paper.

③ AGES AND AGES

Ali, Billi, and Charli are siblings. Four years ago, Billi was two years older than Charli is now, which is in turn three times Ali's current age. Two years ago, Billi was eight times older than Ali. How old is each sibling?

✦ Answer on p.180

BILLI   **CHARLI**   **ALI**

10
24
11

18   17   10   17

✦ Answer on p.180

④ BRAIN CHAINS

Start with the number at the left of each chain, then apply each operation in turn until you reach the "RESULT" link, making a note of your answer. Try to complete each chain without using a calculator or making any written notes.

✦ Answers on p.180

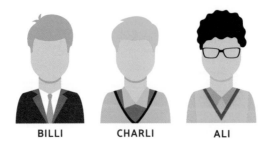

EASY
36 — -14 — ÷11 — +50% — x6 — -50% — RESULT

MEDIUM
20 — -70% — x5 — ÷3 — +61 — -25 — RESULT

HARD
47 — +26 — -7 — $x^{1/2}$ — x7 — $x^{3}/7$ — RESULT

⑤ A QUESTION OF LEGS

There are 23 animals in a field, consisting of a mix of geese and goats. You know that the geese and the goats between them have 76 legs, so how many goats are in the field? Assume that all goats have four legs and all geese have two legs.

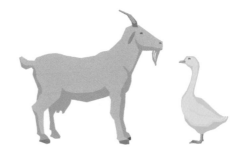

✦ Answer on p.180

⑥ CUBIC COUNTING

How many cubes have been used to build the structure shown? You should assume that all "hidden" cubes are present, and that it started off as a perfect 4×4×4 arrangement of cubes before any cubes were removed. There are no floating cubes.

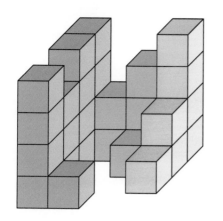

✦ Answer on p.180

⑦ MINI KROPKI

Can you figure out how to place a number from 1 to 9 into each empty square, so no number repeats in the grid? Squares joined by a white dot contain consecutive digits, meaning that they have a numerical difference of 1. Squares joined by a blue dot contain digits where one is exactly twice the value of the other. The absence of a dot means neither relationship applies. Copy the grid out onto a blank piece of paper to keep track of your deductions.

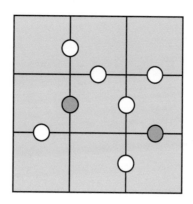

✦ Answer on p.180

⑧ FLOATING NUMBERS

Form each of the three totals below by adding together two or more of the six numbers on the balloons. Each number can be used no more than once per total.

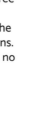

15 25 9 17 16 13

TARGET TOTALS

33 44 66

✦ Answers on p.181

9 PROGENITORIAL PROBLEM

Can you figure out how many granddaughters Mrs. A has? You know that she has:

- Six sons, each with three sisters–all but one of these sons has three daughters, and, furthermore, each of these daughters has two brothers.
- Three daughters, each with two sons of their own, and these sons–Mrs. A's grandsons–each has three sisters.
- One child who has no children of their own.

✦ Answer on p.181

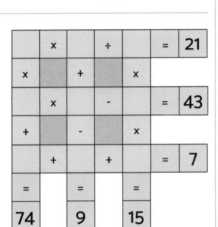

10 ARITHMETIC SQUARE

Figure out how to place the numbers 1 to 9 once each into the nine empty orange squares, so that all of the calculations are correct. Each row and column should result in the given value when the indicated operations are applied. You might find it helpful to copy the puzzle onto a piece of scrap paper first.

✦ Answer on p.181

	x		÷		=	21
x		+		x		
	x		-		=	43
+		-		x		
	+		+		=	7
=		=		=		
74		9		15		

11 A QUESTION OF SPEED

Which of the following vehicles is traveling at the highest average speed?

- A car traveling 6 miles in 15 minutes
- A boat traveling 9 miles in 20 minutes
- A train traveling 26 miles in an hour

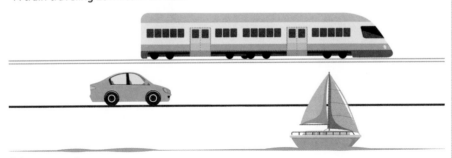

✦ Answer on p.181

12 GRAPE EXPECTATIONS

You buy a bag of grapes and eat half. Your friend then eats one-fifth of what's left. Next, you eat four more grapes each. There are now exactly eight grapes left.

The bag of grapes cost you $2. Assuming this cost is just for the grapes (and not the stalks or the bag they came in) then what is the cost of one grape?

✦ Answer on p.181

13 BAKERY DECISION

If a bag with 3 bagels and 4 doughnuts weighs 344 g, while a bag with 2 bagels and 1 doughnut weighs 136 g, then what would a bag with 1 bagel and 2 doughnuts weigh?

Assume all doughnuts weigh the same, and all bagels weigh the same. You should also assume the bag is of negligible (zero) weight.

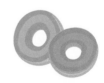

✦ Answer on p.181

(14) PAINTING PROBLEM

Two painters, Mr. A and Miss B, are painting the outside of a house. Working at the same time, it takes them 6 hours to paint the entire front of the house. If Mr. A had been working alone, it would have taken him 8 hours.

Given this information, how long would it have taken Miss B to paint the front of the house alone, assuming that each painter paints at a constant rate?

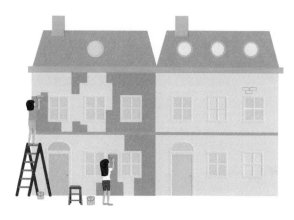

✦ Answer on p.181

(15) BRAIN CHAINS

Start with the number at the top of each building, then apply each operation in turn until you reach the "RESULT" box at ground level, making a note of your answer. Try to complete each entire chain without using a calculator or making any written notes.

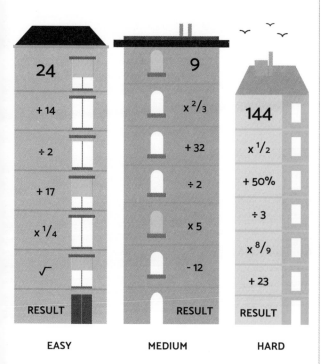

EASY

24
+ 14
÷ 2
+ 17
× 1/4
√
RESULT

MEDIUM

9
× 2/3
+ 32
÷ 2
× 5
- 12
RESULT

HARD

144
× 1/2
+ 50%
÷ 3
× 8/9
+ 23
RESULT

✦ Answer on p.181

(16) HOUSE OF CARDS

If you were to build a house of cards using a regular pack of 52 cards, what is the maximum number of layers you could build? Count both the vertical and flat levels as layers, so, for example, this illustration shows 5 layers. Assume that the bottom layer has to be a "standing up" layer, rather than one of the flat layers.

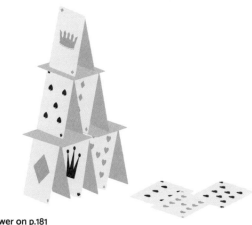

✦ Answer on p.181

How many did you get correct?

1–6: Your mathematical ability would benefit from substantial practice. In chapter 4, focus on activities with the "number skills" calculator icon.

7–12: You have good basic math ability, but could use more practice. Find numerical chapter 4 activities to boost your numeracy.

13–16: Your ability to think clearly while handling numbers is excellent. If you enjoy numerical challenges, stretch yourself further with the calculator-icon activities in chapter 4.

PROBLEM-SOLVING

The ability to think clearly and logically is more of a question of practice than you might think. Tackle these problems by breaking each of them down with a step-by-step process.

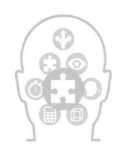

① BIRTHDAY BOGGLER
Matt will be 29 years old next year, even though just two days ago, he was only 26 years old. How can this be possible?

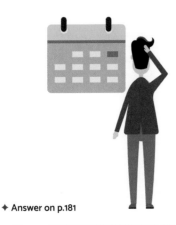

✦ Answer on p.181

② DRINK DIVISION
You have three containers. One holds 2 liters of liquid, one holds 5 liters, and one holds 7 liters. The largest container, the 7-liter one, is full to the brim with water. Assuming that you can pour water between containers without spilling any, how can you measure exactly 6 liters of water? You should not do it "by eye." Each time you pour water between containers you should continue until either the receiving container is full or the pouring container is empty. No water can be discarded or added from elsewhere.

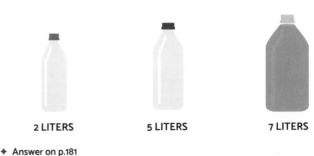

2 LITERS   5 LITERS   7 LITERS

✦ Answer on p.181

③ PATH PROBLEM
Can you find a way of tracing a path through these nine ladybugs so that the path passes through the middle of all nine using just *four* straight lines? You might want to use a ruler or other straight edge to make sure your lines don't bend.

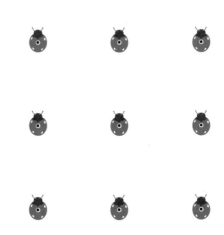

✦ Answer on p.181

4 **A QUESTION OF TRUTH**

Five people are interviewed following a crime, and each gives a different statement. Each ends their statement with a different pronouncement. Which of these people, if any, could be telling you the truth?

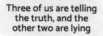
Four of us are telling the truth, and the other one is lying

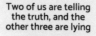
Three of us are telling the truth, and the other two are lying

Two of us are telling the truth, and the other three are lying

One of us is telling the truth, and the other four are lying

All of us are lying

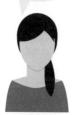
PERSON 1

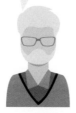
PERSON 2

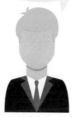
PERSON 3

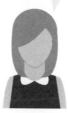
PERSON 4

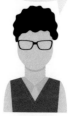
PERSON 5

✦ Answer on p.181

---

5 **CAKE CUTTING**

Imagine that you have a perfectly cylindrical cake, as shown here. How can you divide it into eight identically sized pieces, using just three cuts?

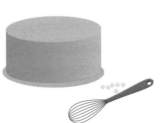

✦ Answer on p.182

---

6 **CARD CONFUSION**

A blind person is handed a normal pack of 52 playing cards and told that 25 of the cards are upside down. They are asked to place the cards into two piles so that each pile has exactly the same number of upside-down cards. How can they do this? The cards feel exactly the same, no matter which way up they are.

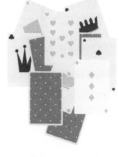

✦ Answer on p.182

---

7 **BOTTLING DILEMMA**

I've agreed to leave exactly half a bottle of juice for my friend, who is a stickler for precision. Assuming that the bottle was full to the brim when I started, how can I be sure I am leaving half of its contents? The bottle has indents at the side and bottom, and is narrower at the top, so standing it up and then doing it "by eye" is not accurate enough.

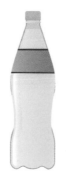

✦ Answer on p.182

---

8 **COIN CHALLENGE**

Imagine that you have four identical coins:

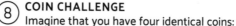

How can you arrange the four coins so that every coin touches *every* other coin simultaneously?

✦ Answer on p.182

⑨ CRATE EXPECTATIONS

You have 12 apples and 3 crates of different sizes. How can you divide those 12 apples among the crates so that each crate holds exactly 6 apples?

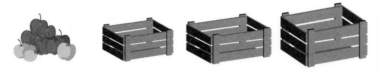

✦ Answer on p.182

⑩ THE BACKWARD PANTS

Imagine that you are wearing a pair of pants, if you are not already so dressed. How can you place your left hand in the right pocket, and your right hand in the left pocket, without crossing your arms?

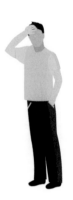

✦ Answer on p.182

⑪ THE BURNING ROPES

You have two ropes, and you know that each takes exactly half an hour to burn from end to end. The ropes, however, burn at variable rates. One might conceivably take 1 minute to burn half of its length, but another 29 minutes to burn the remaining half.

How can you use these two ropes to time exactly 22 minutes and 30 seconds, without needing to guess? Both ends of each rope can be lit, if you like.

✦ Answer on p.182

⑫ THE BOTTLE AND THE BEAN

You are given a glass wine bottle sealed in the traditional way with a cork. Instead of being filled with wine, however, there is instead a solitary bean sitting in the bottom of the bottle.

How can you get the bean out of the bottle, without either smashing the glass or removing the cork from the bottle?

✦ Answer on p.182

⑬ COUNTING CATS

Your neighbor tells you, "All but two of my cats are white, all but two are ginger, and all but two are tortoiseshell." How many cats does your neighbor have?

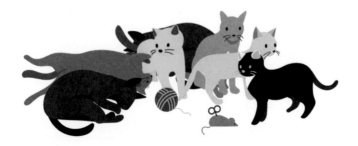

✦ Answer on p.182

⑭ CALENDAR SEARCH

Your friend tells you their birthday is in May, but asks you to tell them the exact date by playing a higher/lower game. Each time you give a date, they will tell you whether that day of the month is correct, too low, or too high. Assuming you suggest dates using an optimal strategy, what is the maximum number of dates you will need to say?

✦ Answer on p.182

15 STEEL AND WATER
You have been given a full glass of water, into which a stainless-steel screw has been dropped. How can you get the screw out of the glass, without spilling the water, touching the glass, or placing anything at all into the water?

✦ Answer on p.182

16 PIZZA PROBLEM
You have a square pizza, of which you have already eaten one-quarter. Four of your friends also want some of the pizza. How can you cut the remaining pizza so that they each receive one piece, and all four of those pieces are exactly the same shape and size?

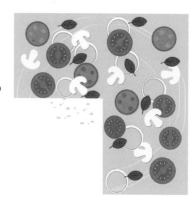

✦ Answer on p.182

17 THE NON-LEAKY BUCKET
Imagine you have a lidless bucket full almost to the brim with water. How can you turn it upside down, and then back the right way up again, without spilling any water? You have only a normal bucket, with the top side completely open and without any lid or other covering.

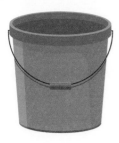

✦ Answer on p.182

How many did you get correct?

1–6: Good job for practicing, but it would be a good idea to find further similar tasks to try. In chapter 4, look out for any activity with the problem-solving (jigsaw piece) icon.

7–13: You have good basic problem-solving ability, but you could use more practice. Try some chapter 4 activities with the jigsaw piece icon.

14–19: Your ability to solve problems is excellent. Maintain your skill using problem-solving activities in chapter 4.

18 UNLIKELY AVERAGES
You're reading a book on world flora when you come across the claim that 75 percent of the world's trees are shorter than average. This surprises you, since shouldn't half the world's trees be smaller than average while the other half be taller than average?

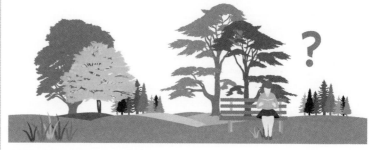

✦ Answer on p.183

19 HOURGLASS DILEMMA
You have two hourglasses, one of which takes 8 minutes for the sand to pass through and the other of which takes 14 minutes for the sand to pass through.

Assuming you have only the hourglasses, and don't want to guess, how can you use them to time a period of 20 minutes?

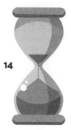

14

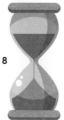

8

✦ Answer on p.183

DECISION-MAKING

We all face real-life problems from time to time, and being able to think rationally about them is critical to making sensible decisions. Test your reasoning skills with these puzzles.

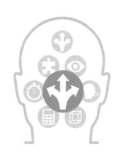

① TRUTH AND LIES
Three people are being questioned. One of them always lies, one of them sometimes lies, and one of them never lies. They each give the following statements: Which person–A, B or C–is the one who never lies?

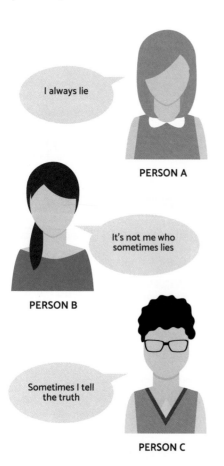

> I always lie

PERSON A

> It's not me who sometimes lies

PERSON B

> Sometimes I tell the truth

PERSON C

② THE BIASED COIN
You need to make a decision by flipping a coin, but the only coin you have on hand is unevenly weighted: when flipped, it lands on one side more often than the other. How can you use this coin to give you a fair decision, with an even chance of either of two options being picked?

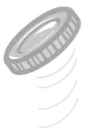

✦ Answer on p.183

③ IF AND ONLY IF
You are friends with two identical twins who you cannot tell apart by sight. However, you know that one of them always lies, while the other one always tells the truth. You meet one of them in the street and ask, "Are we still going to the movies tonight?" They reply:

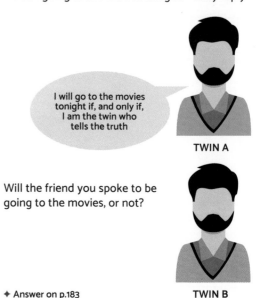

> I will go to the movies tonight if, and only if, I am the twin who tells the truth

TWIN A

Will the friend you spoke to be going to the movies, or not?

TWIN B

✦ Answer on p.183

(4) THE LABELED JARS

You have three jars for condiments, all of which are labeled incorrectly. You need salt but only wish to taste the contents of a single jar in order to find it. Which jar should you taste to be sure of locating the salt?

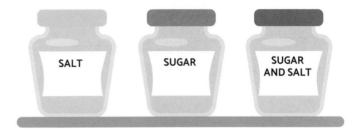

✦ Answer on p.183

(5) DIAMOND DECISION

You are shown three cups and told one of them has a diamond beneath it. You are asked to choose a cup and told that you win the diamond if you choose the cup covering it. You choose a cup. The person showing you the cups knows where the diamond is and turns over one of the two you didn't choose to show you that there's nothing beneath it. They then offer you the chance to change your choice of cup. Should you stick to your decision, or switch?

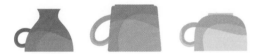

✦ Answer on p.183

(7) SQUASH

You are playing squash with two colleagues, Peter and Paul. They promise that if you can win two games in a row out of the next three, they'll buy you dinner. You will play alternate games against Peter and Paul, but you can choose who to play first. You also know that Paul is more likely to beat you than Peter. Should you play Paul, Peter, then Paul; or Peter, Paul, then Peter?

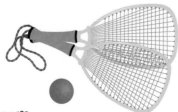

✦ Answer on p.183

(6) ROLL THE DIE

A friend offers you an unusual bet: they will buy you a car if you can roll a six on a regular six-sided die. If you don't roll a six at all, you have to buy them a car. You will be given three chances to roll a six. Is the bet fair?

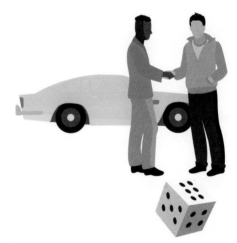

✦ Answer on p.183

How many did you get correct?

0–2: Good job for practicing, but it would be a good idea to find more similar tasks to try.

3–4: You have good basic decision-making ability, but could use more practice..

5–6: You have good logical reasoning skills, so should be capable of making sensible decisions.

ATTENTION AND FOCUS

With so many distractions all around us, it can be difficult truly to pay attention and focus on a task at hand. Practice shutting out the world around you with these puzzles.

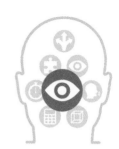

① NUMBER SEARCH
Find all of the listed numbers in the grid. They may be written in any direction, including diagonally, and may read either forward or backward.

6	9	3	6	6	8	5	1	0	7	2	9
1	2	8	9	0	8	5	8	8	8	2	6
1	1	2	6	3	9	7	6	5	3	1	8
4	7	5	8	7	2	0	9	2	7	4	7
2	0	1	8	1	8	6	5	9	1	4	1
1	3	8	1	7	0	8	6	7	2	8	4
6	7	3	4	6	0	8	8	6	4	8	0
3	9	3	9	6	5	6	0	2	7	2	3
0	1	6	8	9	6	6	2	5	3	7	6
9	8	8	0	8	9	9	5	4	1	7	3
6	2	0	9	0	7	3	8	6	8	6	8
8	1	8	7	0	0	7	9	1	2	1	7

11263	71219
1438	79224
27015	85621
33680	85744
37145	86687
60905	86868
70379	89418
70960	96859

✦ Answer on p.183

② CIRCUIT BOARD
Which of the listed pieces, 1 to 4, fits exactly into the gap to complete the circuit board? You may need to rotate, but not flip over, the correct piece.

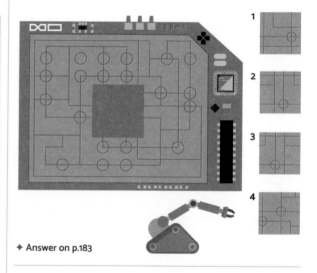

✦ Answer on p.183

③ ODD ONE OUT
Which of these four shapes is the odd one out, and why?

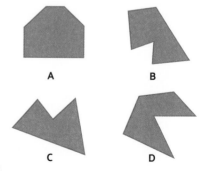

A

B

C

D

✦ Answer on p.183

4 WARP MAZE

Can you find your way through the maze, from the entrance to the exit? When you reach a wormhole you may–if you like–"warp" to any wormhole of the same color. You may also pass over the hole and ignore it.

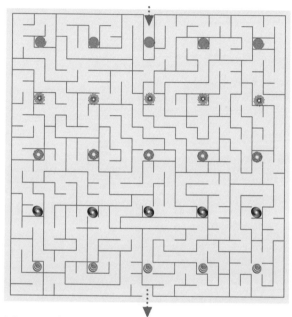

✦ Answer on p.183

6 TWISTING TOTAL

Ignoring any dead-end paths, can you say how many times you need either to turn left or follow a path around to the left as you solve this maze? Start at the top and exit at the bottom. See if you can figure this out without making written notes (and without drawing on the maze).

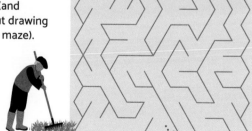

✦ Answer on p.184

5 CUBE CONUNDRUM

If you were to cut out and fold up this shape in order to make a complete six-sided cube, which of the five options below would be the result?

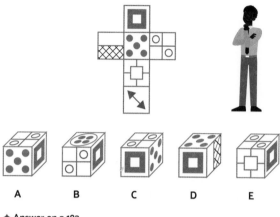

A   B   C   D   E

✦ Answer on p.183

7 MISSING FACE

Which of the five faces shown below should replace the blank face on the left-most cube, so that all three pictures would show different views of the same cube? The face might need to be rotated before being placed.

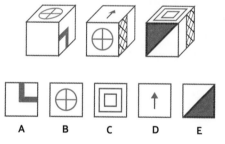

A   B   C   D   E

✦ Answer on p.184

> **How did you find each puzzle? Give yourself a score from 1 (hard) to 3 (easy) for each task.**
>
> **1–7:** You could use more practice, so try some activities in chapter 4 bearing the attention-and-focus (eye) icon.
>
> **8–14:** You have good attention and focus. Do some of the focused tasks in chapter 4 with as few distractions as possible.
>
> **15–21:** You have great attention and focus. To maintain it that way, keep doing some of the attention-demanding activities in chapter 4.

THINKING SPEED AND REACTION TIME

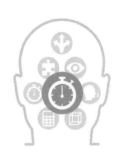

Making quick decisions can be a survival skill, but thinking speed is usually the first cognitive attribute to begin declining with age. How quickly you can solve the puzzles on these two pages?

① MISSING DOMINO

You can form all but one of a regular set of dominoes in this grid. Which domino is missing? Dominoes can be formed by selecting two horizontally or vertically touching squares, as shown by the example shaded in pink. A "o" represents a blank on a traditional domino. Time yourself.

3	3	2	1	6	4	6	5
5	4	5	1	0	0	6	2
0	4	0	2	3	5	5	2
3	4	2	0	3	4	3	2
1	2	4	5	0	1	2	0
6	5	0	1	4	3	5	6
1	1	6	6	5	3	4	1

✦ Answers on p.184

② BRIDGE MAZE

See how quickly you can find your way from the top to the bottom of the maze. You can follow the paths as they pass under the bridges or over the bridges.

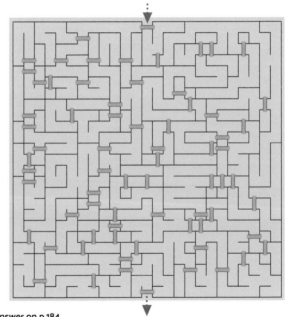

✦ Answer on p.184

③ OUT OF SEQUENCE

Time yourself to see how quickly you can work out which letter is missing from the sequence to the right. When you find the answer, stop the clock.

✦ Answer on p.184

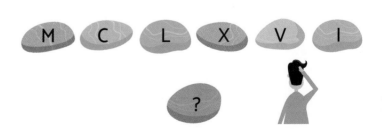

M C L X V I

?

4 SUDOKU ERROR

Imagine overlaying these two grids, so all the blank spaces in one were filled with the numbers from the other, forming a complete sudoku grid. There would be an error in this grid, however, since no number can repeat in any row, column, or colored 3x3 box. Which number should you change, and what to, to create a valid solution? Start a timer and stop it when you find the answer.

✦ Answers on p.184

	6		5		3		4	
4		7		1		8		6
	1		6		8		3	
3		6		9		1		8
	8		3		7		9	
9		4		5		6		3
7		3		8		2		4
	9		4		6		8	
6		8		2		3		9

8		9		7		2		1
	3		9		2		5	
2		5		4		9		7
	5		2		4		7	
1		2		6		4		5
	7		8		1		2	
	2		1		9		6	
5		1		3		7		2
4		7		5		1		

5 COUNTRY INTERSECTION

What two rules have been used to sort the countries in this Venn diagram? The country in the intersection has both rules applied.

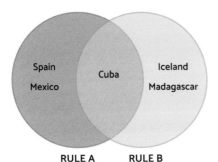

Spain
Mexico
Cuba
Iceland
Madagascar

RULE A   RULE B

✦ Answers on p.184

6 SPOT THE DIFFERENCE

There are five differences between these images. How many can you spot in 1 minute?

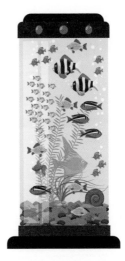
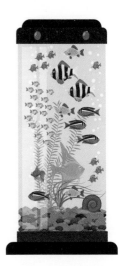

✦ Answers on p.184

7 ODD ONE OUT

How quickly can you identify the odd one out in each line?

1. Indian – Mediterranean – Atlantic – Pacific – Southern

2. Gold – copper – bronze – silver – platinum

3. Banana – strawberry – canary – lemon – daffodil

4. Boxer – Brittany – Pointer – Sphynx – Newfoundland

5. Argentina – Paraguay – Venezuela – Bolivia – Chile

✦ Answers on p.184

How did you find each puzzle? Give yourself a score from 1 (hard) to 3 (easy) for each task.

1–6: You could use more practice, so try the other puzzles in this book and see how quickly you can solve them.

7–12: You have good thinking speed. Try the activities in chapter 4 requiring speed of thought–those with the stopwatch icon.

13–21: You have great thinking speed. Maintain that speed and reaction time with the speedy activities in chapter 4.

SPATIAL VISUALIZATION

The world is 3-D, but we spend much of our lives taking in information from flat pages or screens. Practicing transforming between the two is important, including for map reading.

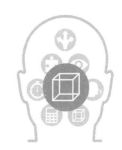

① PYRAMID NETS

Imagine cutting out these shapes and then folding them along the black lines. How many of them could be folded to make complete four-sided pyramids (tetrahedrons)? Which ones?

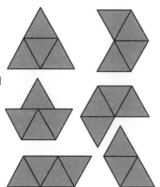

✦ Answer on p.184

② PAPER CUTTING

Pretend that you have a square of paper in front of you, and that you then fold it exactly in half three times in succession. Next, you make a single cut, in one straight line, and end up with the following result:

What three folds did you make, and where was the cut? See if you can figure out a solution in your head, then use an actual piece of paper to test your idea.

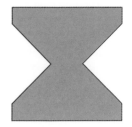

✦ Answer on p.184

③ CUBE NETS

Imagine cutting out these shapes and then folding them along the black lines. Most of them could be folded to make complete 6-sided cubes, except for three. Which three?

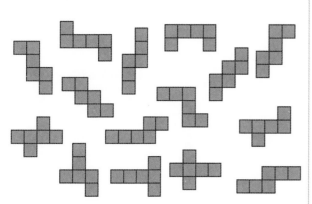

✦ Answer on p.184

④ CUBE NET PATTERN

Without actually cutting anything out, can you say which of these four shapes could be folded to make a cube that exactly matches that shown below?

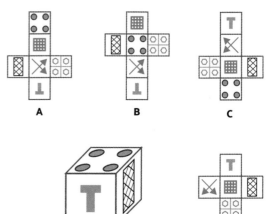

A   B   C

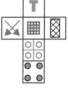

D

✦ Answer on p.184

CUBE VIEW
(5) If you were to view this arrangement of cubes from side on, in the direction shown by the arrow, what would the silhouette look like? Copy out the 5x5 grid, then shade the squares that would be occupied by a cube. An example is given, to show how it works.

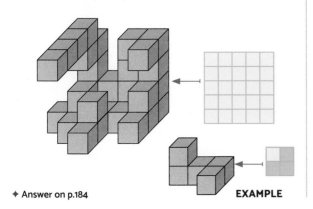

EXAMPLE

✦ Answer on p.184

ROTATED CUBES
(6) Each of the following arrangements of cubes is viewed from a different angle. Three of the arrangements are identical, but one is different. Which one?

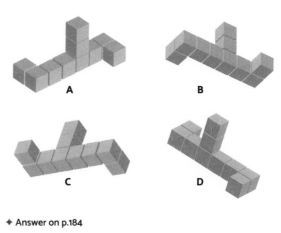

A

B

C

D

✦ Answer on p.184

ROUTE MASTER
(7) You are standing in the square marked with the red arrow, facing in the direction shown. Which of the following three sets of instructions will take you from this square to one of the three houses? Which house? For a bonus, which of the dangerous holes do each of the two incorrect routes end up at?

⬆ means "travel forward 1 square"

➡ means "stay in the same square but turn to face 90 degrees to your right"

⬅ means "stay in the same square but turn to face 90 degrees to your left"

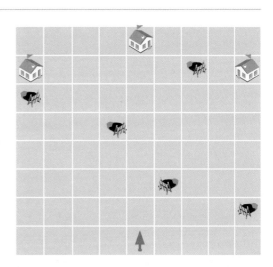

⬆⬆⬅⬆➡⬆➡⬆⬆⬅⬆⬆➡⬆
⬆⬆⬅⬆⬆⬆➡⬆➡⬆⬆⬆⬅➡⬆

INSTRUCTIONS 1

⬅⬆⬆⬆⬆➡⬆⬆⬆⬆⬆⬆➡⬆⬆⬆
➡⬆⬆⬅⬆⬆⬆➡⬆⬆⬆➡⬆⬆➡⬆

INSTRUCTIONS 2

➡⬆⬆⬆⬅⬆⬆➡⬆⬅⬆⬆⬆⬅➡⬆➡⬆⬆
⬅⬆⬆⬅⬆⬆⬆⬆⬅⬆➡⬆➡⬆⬆⬆➡⬆⬆⬆⬆
⬆⬆➡➡⬆⬆⬆⬆➡⬆⬆⬆➡⬅⬆⬆⬆⬅⬆⬆⬆⬆

INSTRUCTIONS 3

✦ Answers on p.184

How many did you get correct?

0–2: Try copying out some of the pyramid or cube nets, then cut and fold them by hand to see how they work. Look for activities in chapter 4 with the spatial visualization (cube) icon. These are good for spatial awareness and orientation, too.

3–5: You have good basic visualization skills, but try practicing giving map directions to build your abilities..

5–7: You have great visualization skills.

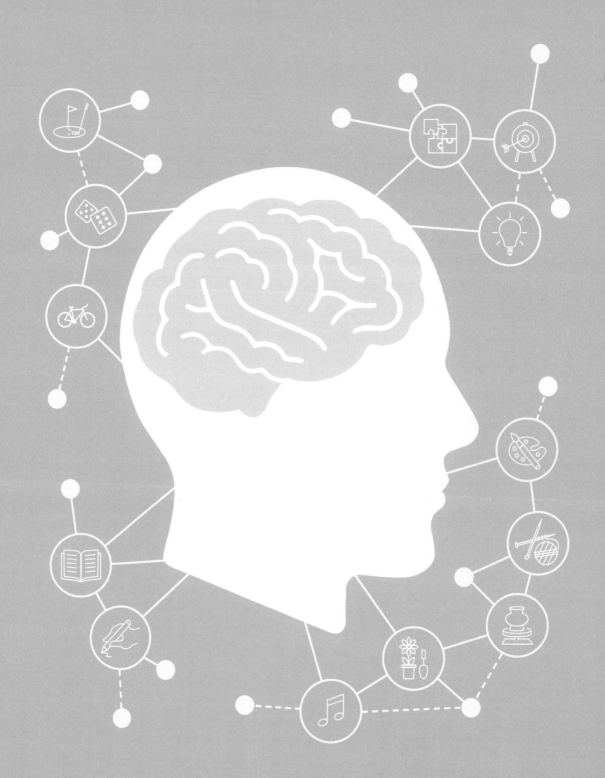

TRY NEW THINGS

THE BENEFITS OF LEARNING NEW THINGS

To keep your brain young, you need to keep trying new things–whatever your age. From drawing to dancing, there are dozens of pleasurable and challenging ways of keeping your brain active.

CRAFTS AND HOBBIES (pp.116–155)
Trying your hand at a new craft or hobby can be very fulfilling, because it often involves creating something. Consider drawing, pottery, or origami, birdwatching, or stargazing.

READY, SET, GO!

The desire to learn something new and the satisfaction of doing so are themselves important brain boosters because they generate dopamine and serotonin–neurotransmitters that activate brain cells and make you feel good. Mind-stretching activities can be physical or sensual–they don't have to be purely intellectual. The main thing is to do it, enjoy it, and do it again. Remember, though, that practicing most things only gets you nearer to perfection at that particular thing. To improve your all-around mental abilities, you need to keep taking on new challenges, giving your brain the equivalent of a workout at the gym for your muscles.

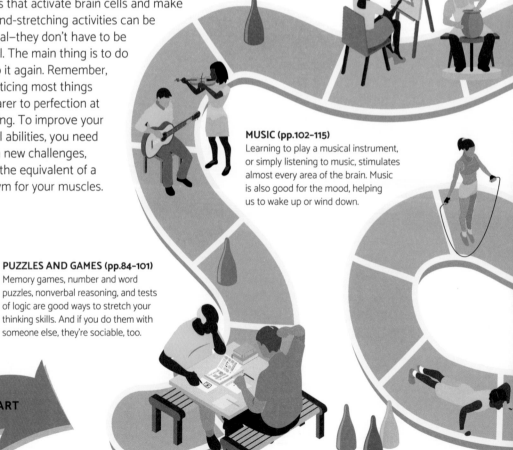

MUSIC (pp.102–115)
Learning to play a musical instrument, or simply listening to music, stimulates almost every area of the brain. Music is also good for the mood, helping us to wake up or wind down.

PUZZLES AND GAMES (pp.84–101)
Memory games, number and word puzzles, nonverbal reasoning, and tests of logic are good ways to stretch your thinking skills. And if you do them with someone else, they're sociable, too.

START

A REWARDING RETIREMENT

Retirement may sound like bliss, but one survey of 1,000 recently retired people found that, on average, they became bored within a year of stopping paid employment. If you enjoy your work and can do it as well as you ever could, don't stop! But if your work has started to bore or exhaust you, retirement offers an opportunity to take up new interests and learn new things—and exercise your brain while doing so.

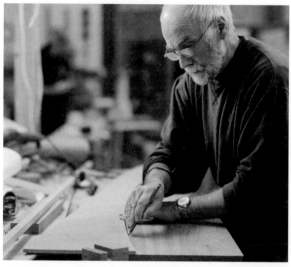

SPORTS (pp.156–169)
Exercise makes us feel great, and a short walk is enough to get the brain whirring. Sports such as golf, tennis, yoga, and dancing are a good way to have fun and meet like-minded people.

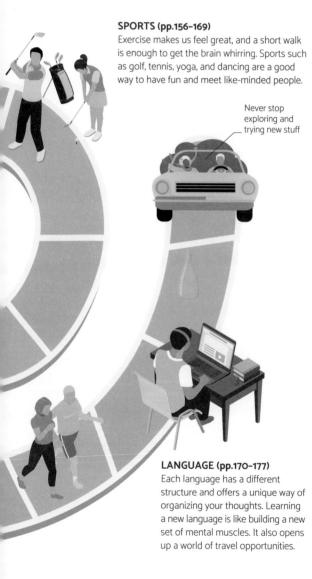

Never stop exploring and trying new stuff

CHOICES, CHOICES
After years of being driven by the demands of a job, it can be difficult to choose what to do in retirement. Popular pastimes include arts and crafts (such as woodworking), country walks, cooking, and wine tasting.

> **Retired people have, on average, seven and a half hours of leisure time every day**

LANGUAGE (pp.170–177)
Each language has a different structure and offers a unique way of organizing your thoughts. Learning a new language is like building a new set of mental muscles. It also opens up a world of travel opportunities.

BRAIN-TRAINING GAMES
The thousands of "brain-training" games available promise to make your brain work better, yet it is not clear that they do. Different parts of the brain do different things, so a task that challenges one brain function, such as remembering lots of objects, may well make you better at that, but not necessarily better at anything else. If you enjoy playing these games, play on! But if you want to improve your general cognitive skills, it's better to try an activity that involves dealing with others, interacting physically with objects, and exercising your limbs as well as doing a mental task.

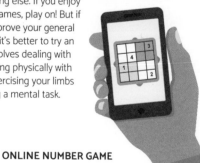

ONLINE NUMBER GAME

SOCIAL ACTIVITIES

Maintaining close friendships and an active social life
is one of the most important things you can do
to keep your brain fit.

A daily phone call to someone who is isolated may keep both of you from feeling lonely

STAY SOCIAL

Most people enjoy an active social life when they are young and energetic, but find that their social network shrinks as they get older. Millions of elderly people report that they regularly go for weeks without speaking to another person. But if your friends are distant and your family is busy, how can you forge new friendships and find meaningful social activity? The Global Council on Brain Health has suggested 12 ways to achieve this.

Concentrate on the relationships or social activities you like best

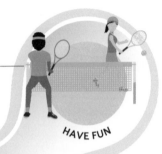

HAVE FUN

ASK FOR HELP

Banish loneliness by making a new connection, reigniting an old friendship, or seeking different opportunities to interact with others

Build and maintain a network of friends, family, or neighbors who you can talk to regularly or ask for help. Try to have at least one person you can confide in

If no one you know can help you to make social connections, talk to a professional–for example, via a telephone hotline, drop-in center, or local religious center

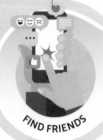

FIND FRIENDS

BUILD BONDS

Being married can be good for brain health, but try also to nurture other important relationships so you have a good support network

If you struggle to get around, or feel unsafe, try to find someone you can ask for help, and who can help you to engage with others

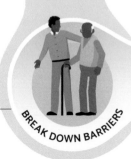

BREAK DOWN BARRIERS

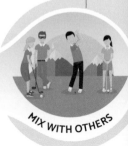

MIX WITH OTHERS

YOUNG AND OLD

Historically, older people played an integral role in the development of young people's lives, and for good reason–mixing with those of another generation is beneficial to young and old alike. Young people help their seniors to understand new things, such as the latest technology, while older people can help younger ones to learn from the wisdom they have accumulated. And as time is more plentiful at both ends of life, young and old are often well suited to spending this time together.

If you are already sociable, try something different. You could join or set up a new group that those in your community would also enjoy

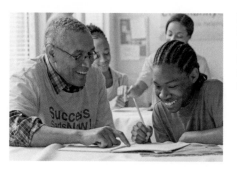

LIVE IN THE MOMENT
Mentoring young people is a good way to be social and keep busy, and you may find that you learn as much from someone you mentor as they learn from you.

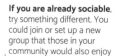

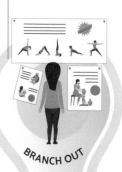

BRANCH OUT

Spend time with people of all ages, including young people. Pass on skills and knowledge to grandchildren, or offer to help at a local community center

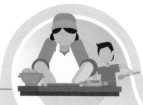

SHARE SKILLS

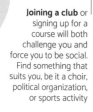

FIND A HOBBY

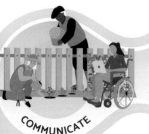

COMMUNICATE

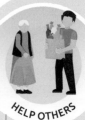

HELP OTHERS

BUMP INTO PEOPLE

Joining a club or signing up for a course will both challenge you and force you to be social. Find something that suits you, be it a choir, political organization, or sports activity

Keep in touch with neighbors, friends, and relatives–try to talk to them regularly in person, on the phone, or by email or another messaging service

Volunteering is a good way to help and engage with others, as is visiting a lonely neighbor and shopping for them, or helping them with cooking or gardening

Find new ways to interact with others by putting yourself in everyday contexts (such as the park or stores) where it's easy to meet new people

MEMORY CHALLENGES

Like the memory tests on pages 56–59, these challenges exercise your working memory (see p.18)–the memory you use to hold information in the short term for immediate use.

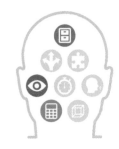

THINKING SKILLS

Train your working memory by practicing observation and attentiveness

•

Improve your focus by filtering out distractions

CHALLENGE 1 | KIM'S GAME

You can train and improve your working memory, and exercises like Kim's Game are used in military training to hone observational skills. The name comes from Rudyard Kipling's book *Kim*, in which the titular character is faced with a similar challenge. Try it by starting with the tray on the left. Take 60 seconds to memorize the items pictured, then cover the image and see how many of the 15 you can recall. The harder levels include duplicates of items and items in different colors, challenging you to recall item, number, and color.

 EASY

 MEDIUM

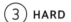 **HARD**

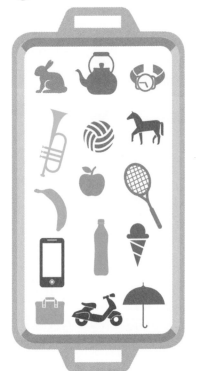

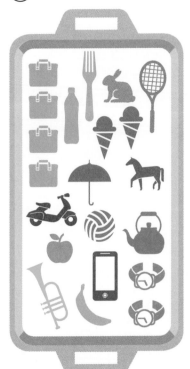

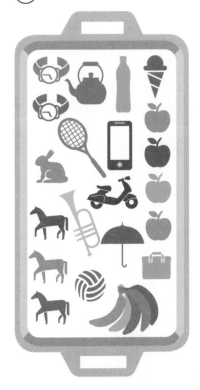

CHALLENGE 2 | GRID MEMORY

For each puzzle, pick one of the two patterns and then study it for as long as you feel you need to memorize it. Then cover it up and try to reproduce it on another piece of paper as accurately as you can. Once you are done, repeat with the other pattern.

1 EASY

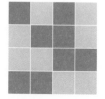 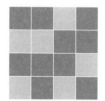

2 MEDIUM

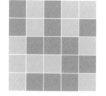 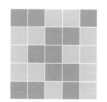

3 HARD

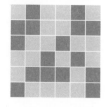 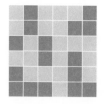

CHALLENGE 3 | MATH MEMORY

First, cover the numbers in purple for the puzzle you are tackling. Then, look at the numbers in green and spend as long as you need memorizing them. Cover the numbers in green and reveal the associated numbers in purple. Which of these numbers can you form by adding two or more of the green numbers you have memorized? There is always at least one valid answer, but there may be more than one.

1 EASY

◆ Answers on p.185

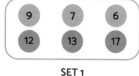 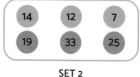

SET 1   SET 2

2 MEDIUM

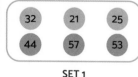 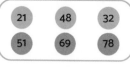

SET 1   SET 2

3 HARD

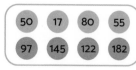 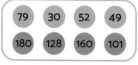

SET 1   SET 2

TAKE IT FURTHER

Working memory, such as that used in the exercises above, is about being attentive, and the ability to filter out unwanted information to focus on the task. If you want to preserve information for longer, many further techniques can help. They work by organizing information, as in the case of mind maps (right), or "chunking" it into memorable morsels and linking it to more memorable information—see pp.86–91.

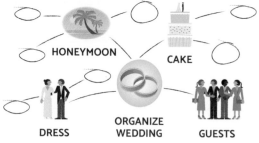

MIND MAP
You can organize information to make it memorable by constructing a network of associated connections called a mind web, or map.

MEMORY TIPS

You can improve your ability to remember specific information using memory-boosting techniques. Try a few different options and see which work best for you.

REMEMBERING NAMES

When you meet someone new, failing to recall their name immediately is very common, because our brains process faces much better than names. When you meet a new person, linking their name with some existing knowledge will mean that you are more likely to recall their name the next time you meet.

① **ANIMALS**
Does the person remind you of an animal? If so, link their name to the animal–the more bizarre the better.

If you meet Amy, and she has very big eyes...

... you might think of an owl, so link the name "Amy" with an image of an owl in your mind.

② **TRY IT OUT**
Watch a new TV show and try to learn some of the characters' names. What animals might you link with their names to help remember?

① **CELEBRITIES**
Can you think of a well-known person with the same name? Link your new acquaintance with that celebrity's features.

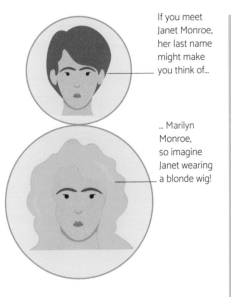

If you meet Janet Monroe, her last name might make you think of...

... Marilyn Monroe, so imagine Janet wearing a blonde wig!

② **TRY IT OUT**
Look at a news story to find some people you do not know. Try thinking of celebrities with similar names and link them to the new names.

ACRONYMS

Acronyms are formed by taking the first letter from several words to form a new word. The best acronyms link with their subject. Some contrivance is often required, but this may also help you to remember the words. For example, the UK's Home Office Large Major Enquiry System (a police computer program) is known as HOLMES, named after Sherlock Holmes.

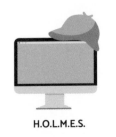

H.O.L.M.E.S.

MEMORY PEGS

The most common mnemonic system (a technique to help you remember) establishes a sequence of familiar "pegs." The pegs are easily visualized words that you learn and associate with a number, letter, or anything with a sequence that you will not forget. This will help you to remember things in a particular order. Once you have established your pegs, you can link, or "hang," new information on each one.

(1) **ESTABLISH YOUR PEGS**
It can be useful if your memorable sequence (numbers, for example) rhymes with your pegs. If the pegs rhyme, they are more likely to stick in your mind. Take some time to see if you can remember these rhyming number pegs or memorize your own set.

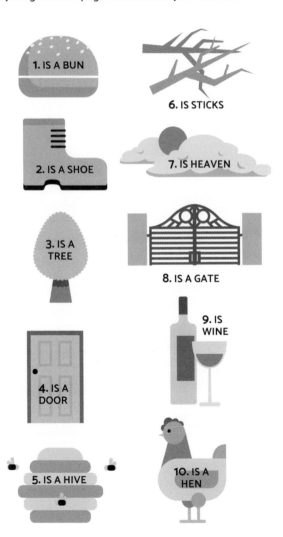

1. IS A BUN

6. IS STICKS

2. IS A SHOE

7. IS HEAVEN

3. IS A TREE

8. IS A GATE

4. IS A DOOR

9. IS WINE

5. IS A HIVE

10. IS A HEN

(2) **HANG ITEMS ON YOUR PEGS**
Hang the information you want to remember onto your pegs. Visualize your peg and the thing you need to remember—such as the ingredients in a recipe—together in the most bizarre way possible.

If you were memorizing cake ingredients, you could think of a bag of **sugar** wearing the first peg (a **bun**) as a hat!

For the second ingredient and peg, you might imagine stepping in **butter** and having to clean it off your **shoe**.

To remember the eggs on the "three" peg, how about imagining lots of **eggs** growing on the **tree**?

For the fourth and final ingredient, you might imagine the mess it would make if you threw a bag of **flour** at the **door**.

(3) **TRY IT OUT**
Write a short shopping list. Take the pegs you memorized and attach the shopping items to your pegs. How many items from the list can you remember?

ACROSTICS

For acrostics, you take the first letter of each word you want to remember and then turn the letters into new words that share the same first letters. The name "Roy G. Biv," for example, is an acrostic to remember the colors of the rainbow.

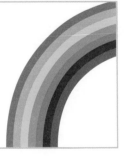

TRY STORY CONSTRUCTION

Stories come naturally to people, and storing information in a narrative structure makes it much easier to remember.

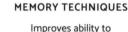

MEMORY TECHNIQUES

Improves ability to remember things

•

Create scenes and stories to remember new information

Use rhyme to improve your recall ability

MAKING A SCENE

In the event that you need to remember a set of random words, visualizing the words as a scene will make them much easier to remember. People can remember more than 2,000 pictures with at least 90 percent accuracy in recognition tests over a period of several days. This excellent memory for pictures consistently exceeds our ability to remember words.

1 PICTURE THIS
If you needed to remember the words: candle, moon, hat, ship, and stripe, you could use them to create a scene. The more weird the scene is, the easier it will be to remember.

2 TRY IT OUT
Remember the following list of words (or your own list) by making a scene like the one here. Memorize these words: table, flower, wheel, helmet, diary.

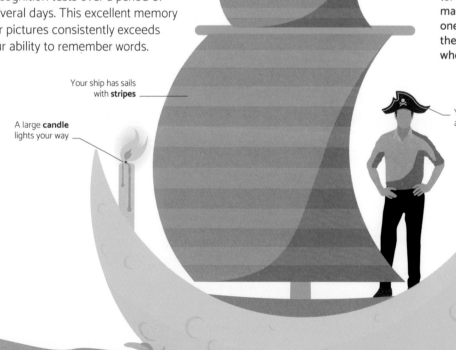

Your ship has sails with **stripes**

A large **candle** lights your way

You are wearing a pirate **hat**

You are traveling on the **moon** as your **ship**

TELLING A TALE

Creating a story is useful if the things you need to remember must be recalled in a particular order, and is even more useful if the words are not that familiar. Your story still needs to be bizarre, but it must also have a certain logic to it, so that the sequence of events unfolds naturally in the right order.

① VISUALIZING THE WORDS

Imagine you had to remember the hierarchy of living things: Kingdom, Phylum, Class, Order, Family, Genus, Species. Each word can be visualized as something, even if it is not an exact match.

KINGDOM
You might imagine a big map showing a fairy-tale **kingdom**, with a crown in the middle.

PHYLUM
Phylum sounds like "film," so you imagine zooming into the map as if it were the start of a **film**.

CLASS
The story takes you into a classroom where a **class** of children is being taught.

ORDER
Some of the class is being disruptive, and the teacher is struggling to keep **order**.

FAMILY
The disruption is being caused by two pupils who are from the same **family**.

GENUS
The two students have been told by their parents that they are **geniuses** (close enough to "Genus").

SPECIES
The two children are convinced that they are geniuses, and so keep making **speeches!**

② TRY IT OUT

Try to memorize the planets of our solar system: Mercury, Venus, Earth, Mars, Jupiter, Saturn, Uranus, Neptune. Visualize each word as a concrete thing.

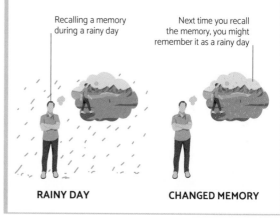

BEWARE THE CHANGING MEMORY!

Accurate recall of events is surprisingly rare. If it is important that you remember something that happens to you (for example, if you witness a crime) it is best to write it down as soon as you possibly can, including every detail. This is because memories are constantly changing. If you recalled a hike on a sunny day at another time when it was raining, there is a chance that the rain during the time you recalled the memory may attach itself to the memory, and next time you might recall the memory as a hike in the rain!

Recalling a memory during a rainy day

Next time you recall the memory, you might remember it as a rainy day

RAINY DAY　　　**CHANGED MEMORY**

RHYME IS NOT CRIME

To make your memory stories even more memorable, try turning them into rhyming poetry. Like the stories, the more ridiculous the poem is, the better. Rhymes are easily recalled because they engage the areas of the brain that deal with rhythm and melody, as well as sound and meaning.

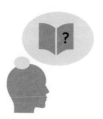 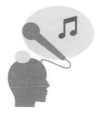 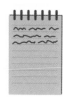

PLAIN WORDS
Many people find it difficult to memorize a block of information straight from a book simply by reading it.

SONG LYRICS
Lots of people find that they remember song lyrics more easily than words they have read from a book.

TRY IT OUT
Make a list of jobs you need to do. Turn them into rhyming poetry and see how many you remember.

TRY THE MEMORY PALACE

A memory palace is an imaginary place where you plant things that you want to remember. It is particularly useful if you are trying to memorize a number of items in order.

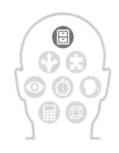

MEMORY TECHNIQUES

Improves ability to remember things

•

Use a place you know well to remember new information

•

Improves ability to recall information in a specific order

BUILDING YOUR PALACE

You could build your own memory palace either by constructing a fantasy house or garden, or by familiarizing yourself with a real place. Sometimes the best memory palaces are actually the places you already know really well, like your own house or maybe the route you take to work.

KNOW YOUR PLACE
Memorize your chosen place so well that when you close your eyes you can conjure up almost every detail, and imagine your walk around it. Do this at least once a day.

Decide on a specific route around your palace; this will always stay the same

Note some permanent landmarks along the way, for example, the lights, a fireplace, and the kitchen sink

Repeat the route in your memory until the steps you take are automatic and the landmarks "leap out" at you

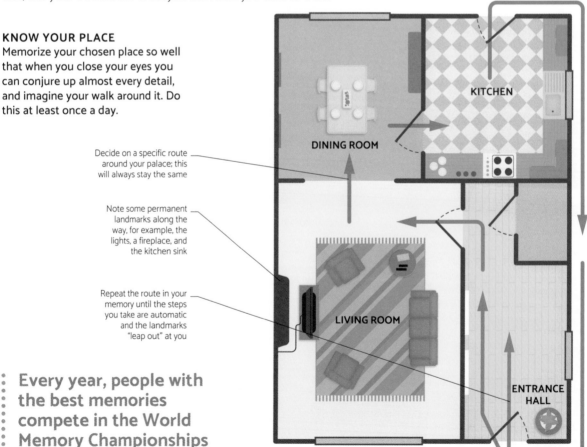

KITCHEN

DINING ROOM

LIVING ROOM

ENTRANCE HALL

Every year, people with the best memories compete in the World Memory Championships

PUTTING THE PALACE TO USE

Note down the things that you want to remember and the order in which you want to use them. Visualize each item as vividly as possible and place it into your memory palace. If it is something that does not have a fixed form, find a way of representing it visually. For example, if you want to make a speech about finance and you want to remember to mention inflation, think of it as a balloon getting bigger and bigger. The more bizarre and attention-grabbing the image, the better.

MEMORY PALACE TECHNIQUE

The memory palace technique (also called the Method of loci, or the Journey Method) is credited by some to Simonides of Ceos, a Greek poet. He was at a dinner when the building collapsed and he was the only survivor. Everyone who died had been buried, but Simonides could identify the dead by remembering where they had been sitting.

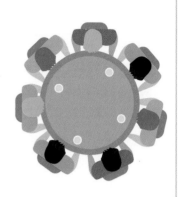

FILLING THE PALACE

If you wanted to remember the three main contributors to climate change (fossil fuels, deforestation, and agriculture) for a speech, you would visualize these things and place them in your palace.

(1) **FOSSIL FUELS**
You open the front door to the smoke coming from a coal barbeque that is blazing away in the hallway.

(2) **DEFORESTATION**
Moving into the living room, you find a man with a chain saw who has felled a tree and is now chopping up your sofa.

(3) **AGRICULTURE**
You get to the dining room and find a cow at your dining table eating a meal with a knife and fork.

(4) **TRY IT OUT**
Write a list of items to pack for a day out and then place them in your memory palace to remember.

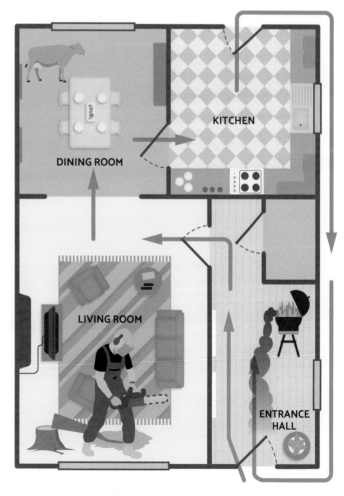

TRY NUMBER PUZZLES

Mathematically minded people love seeing patterns and solving numerical puzzles. Even if you are not one of those people, you might recognize that you need practice at this kind of challenge.

CHALLENGE 1 |
NUMBER PYRAMIDS

Complete each number pyramid by writing a number in each empty brick, so that each brick contains a value equal to the sum of the two bricks immediately beneath it. You may want to copy out each pyramid first.

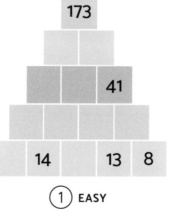

1 EASY

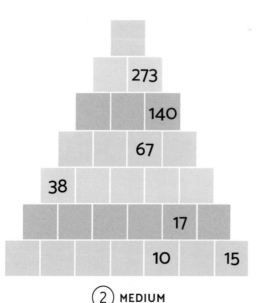

2 MEDIUM

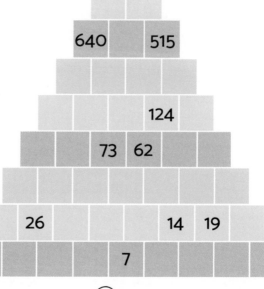

3 HARD

✦ Answers on p.185

CHALLENGE 2 | DIAGONAL DIGITS

For each puzzle, place a digit from 1 to 4, 6, or 7 (depending on the size of the grid) into each square, so that no digit repeats in any row or column. Values outside the grid give the total of the numbers in their indicated diagonal. You may want to copy out each grid first.

Be imaginitive with math—try to see the problem in different ways

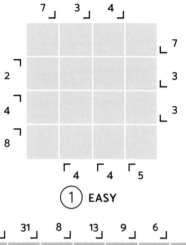

① EASY

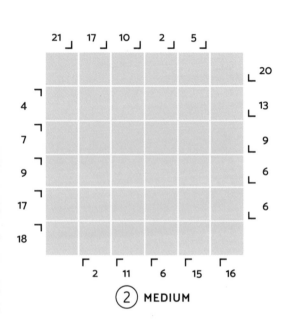

② MEDIUM

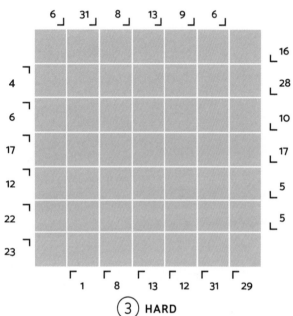

③ HARD

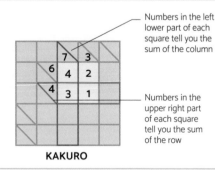

TAKE IT FURTHER

To exercise your numerical brain, stop relying on a calculator or other technology. Use every opportunity to solve life's number problems manually. If that is not enough, puzzle fans can find whole classes of brainteaser based on numerical reasoning. Kakuro requires both arithmetical skill and deductive logic.

Numbers in the left lower part of each square tell you the sum of the column

Numbers in the upper right part of each square tell you the sum of the row

KAKURO

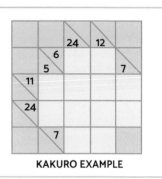

KAKURO EXAMPLE

✦ Answers on p. 185

TRY WORD PUZZLES

As you mature, your language ability becomes crystallized, meaning your knowledge is likely to stay with you. Word games are fun, though, and engaging in wordplay will ensure that your verbal dexterity does not fade.

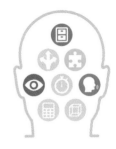

THINKING SKILLS

Bolster your vocabulary memory banks

•

Aid focus

•

Exercise your verbal fluency, giving you precision in thinking about complex things

CHALLENGE 1 | **LETTER SOUP**

Can you rearrange each of these groups of letters to create sets of related words? In each case, every letter must be used once, and no letters should be left over. For each set, the topic and the number of words to find is given.

① **EASY**
Three sports

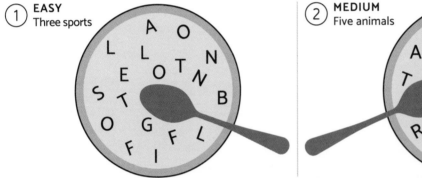

② **MEDIUM**
Five animals

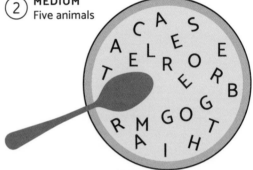

③ **HARD**
Six chemical elements

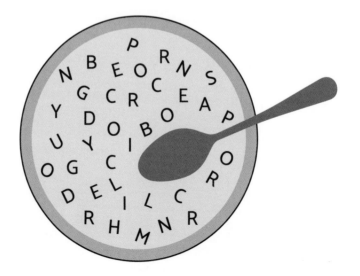

✦ Answers on page 185

CHALLENGE 2 |
PATHFINDER

Can you find a set of related words in each of these three grids? In each grid you should start on the circled letter and then find a path that visits every grid square exactly once, spelling out each of the words as it travels around the grid. The path can travel only horizontally or vertically between squares and cannot skip over or revisit any squares. In the first puzzle, the starting word is highlighted to show how it works.

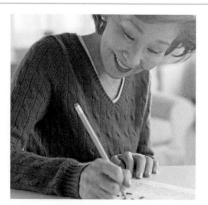

TAKE IT FURTHER

Games and exercises such as solving anagrams, rebuses, and crosswords maintain your verbal aptitude. Mix and match the games to give yourself a more holistic workout. Another way to exercise your ability with words is to read more. Stretch yourself with challenging material, such as a classic novel or poem that will introduce you to new words and different styles of writing and original ways of thinking.

CROSSWORD PUZZLE

① EASY
Colors

```
W  H  I  T  Y  W  R
O  E  T  E  E  O  E
R  A  O  L  L  L  D
G  N  I  E  U  L  B
E  N  V  I  I  N  K
B  W  D  N  P  R  G
R  O  I  G  O  A  Y
```

② MEDIUM
Countries

```
A  N  A  C  U  S  T  R  A
R  I  T  A  A  A  R  B  Z
G  E  N  N  A  L  I  A  I
M  A  C  A  D  N  A  P  L
B  O  D  N  A  T  H  A  J
I  D  P  O  L  I  A  S  M
A  I  A  R  T  U  R  A  E
T  N  A  L  A  G  U  I  X
A  N  Z  H  O  N  D  C  O
```

③ HARD
Flowers

```
S  U  N  F  O  D  E  R  B  U  T  T
E  W  F  F  A  I  G  Y  E  B  R  E
R  O  L  P  D  L  P  P  R  A  C  U
G  L  L  I  Z  A  O  D  N  A  D  P
D  A  U  T  A  A  P  E  S  G  A  R
I  R  C  D  L  E  I  L  I  N  E  D
O  O  H  I  S  N  O  L  L  I  A  S
L  A  I  E  W  A  R  Y  D  W  O  N
U  S  S  E  T  M  A  O  R  S  Y  C
Y  H  E  E  W  A  M  P  A  N  R  A
A  N  T  R  I  I  A  D  P  A  N  N
C  I  H  F  L  L  I  S  Y  T  I  O
```

> **The average person's active vocabulary (words they use) is 10,000–20,000 words, although the total number of words they know might be double this**

✦ Answers on page 185

TRY NONVERBAL REASONING

Also known as abstract reasoning, nonverbal reasoning involves solving problems presented in diagram or picture form, so visual clues, rather than words or numbers, are the basis of the task.

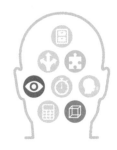

THINKING SKILLS

Tests spatial understanding and awareness

Exercises your skills in solving problems without words

Focuses attention and helps you practice filtering out distractions

CHALLENGE 1 | ODD CUBE OUT

For each puzzle, if you were to cut out and fold up the shape in order to make a complete six-sided cube, which of the four options would result?

(1) **EASY**

A   B    C   D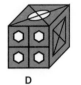

(2) **MEDIUM**

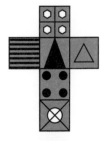
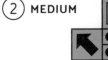

A   B   C   D

(3) **HARD**

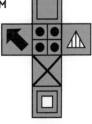

A 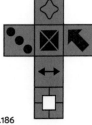   B    C    D

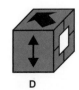

✦ Answers on p.186

CHALLENGE 2 | VISUAL TRANSFORMATION

For each puzzle, which one of the five potential solutions (A–E) should go in the empty box? Use the three completed transformations to figure out what rule or rules are being applied.

✦ Answers on p.186

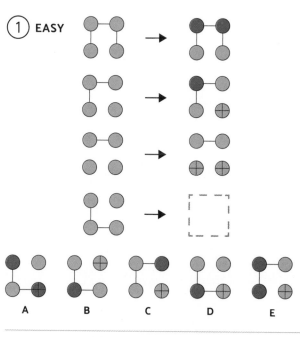

① **EASY**

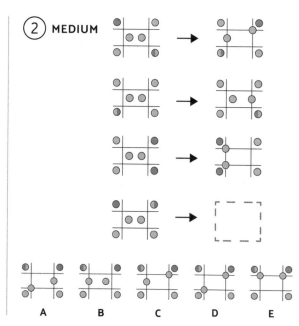

② **MEDIUM**

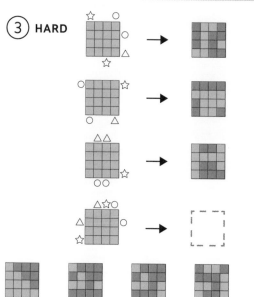

③ **HARD**

If you're curious, take an online IQ test–these tests include nonverbal reasoning tasks, but how accurately they measure "intelligence" is debatable

TAKE IT FURTHER

You may encounter nonverbal reasoning tests throughout life, because they can be used in school entrance exams, in IQ tests, and sometimes even in job interviews. Nonverbal reasoning shows skills that are not limited by words and language, so if you have dyslexia, for instance, or another difficulty in communicating verbally, you can still exercise and demonstrate your other mental skills. Nonverbal reasoning is useful in science, math, engineering, computing, and design.

TRY LOGIC PUZZLES

Some puzzles that use numbers seem to be exercises in numeracy. Sudoku is a popular example, but the numbers are incidental—any set of nine items can be substituted and the puzzle will work just the same. Sudoku is an example of a logical reasoning puzzle.

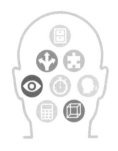

THINKING SKILLS

Test problem-solving abilities with logical reasoning

Improve focus, if you can filter out distractions

CHALLENGE 1 | SUDOKU

This is a completed sudoku grid to show you the rules. The puzzles below have empty squares to be filled up like this, by logical deduction. In each puzzle, place a digit from 1 to 9 into each empty square, so that no digit repeats in any row, column, or bold-lined 3x3 box. Copy out each grid first.

2	5	7	4	8	1	9	6	3
1	9	3	6	2	7	5	4	8
8	4	6	5	3	9	1	7	2
3	6	1	7	5	8	2	9	4
9	8	5	1	4	2	7	3	6
7	2	4	9	6	3	8	5	1
6	3	2	8	7	5	4	1	9
4	7	9	2	1	6	3	8	5
5	1	8	3	9	4	6	2	7

Every row contains the digits 1–9

Every column contains the digits 1–9

Every bold-outlined square must also contain only one instance of every digit

(1) EASY

			6	5	2			
		5				9		
	6	2	3		8	4	1	
5		6	1		9	3		2
4								1
2		8	5		4	6		9
	8	7	9		3	5	6	
		4				2		
			4	6	5			

(2) MEDIUM

	7	4		1	2			
1	6	2		9	8	4		
5	4	8		2	1	7		
7	1	3		6	9	5		
4	3	1		5	7	9		
	5	6		8	3			

(3) HARD

		4	3		9	8		
	9			2			4	
7								9
6			8		2			4
	7					5		
2			7		6			1
4								7
	5			4			6	
		9	6		1	4		

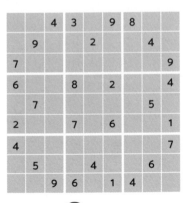

◆ Answers on p.186

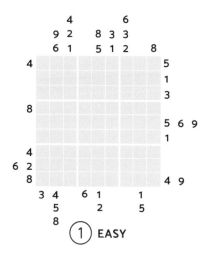

① EASY

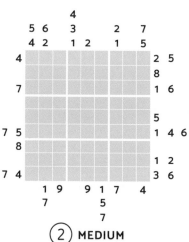

② MEDIUM

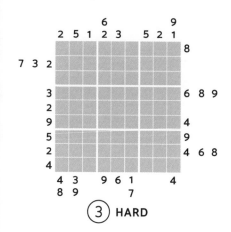

③ HARD

CHALLENGE 2 | OUTSIDE SUDOKU

This is one of many variations on sudoku rules. For each puzzle, place a digit from 1 to 9 into each square, so that no digit repeats in any row, column, or bold-lined 3×3 box. All of the digits outside the grid must be placed into one of the three nearest squares in that digit's row or column. Copy out each grid first.

TAKE IT FURTHER

Experienced sudoku players pick up techniques that make them quicker at solving the puzzles. But don't let the game get stale and repetitive–if sudoku becomes automatic, look for a new challenge. Try sudoku without numbers, 3-D sudoku, and the many other variations with altered rules.

NON-NUMERICAL SUDOKU

Sudoku without numbers can be trickier, because the set of nine items that completes the grid is not as easy to remember as nine digits.

Each stationery item must appear only once in each row, column, and 3x3 grid

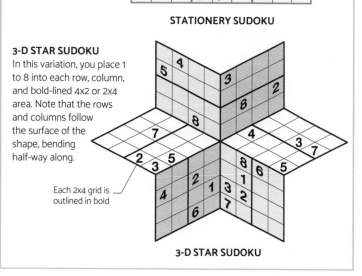

STATIONERY SUDOKU

3-D STAR SUDOKU

In this variation, you place 1 to 8 into each row, column, and bold-lined 4x2 or 2x4 area. Note that the rows and columns follow the surface of the shape, bending half-way along.

Each 2x4 grid is outlined in bold

3-D STAR SUDOKU

✦ Answers on p.186

TRY CREATIVE REASONING PUZZLES

Creative reasoning skills have a wide variety of applications in the real world, from DIY home improvement to wilderness survival, so there are plenty of good reasons to keep practicing them.

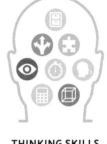

THINKING SKILLS

Encourage experiments in lateral thinking

•

Force you to solve problems in inventive ways

•

May often involve spatial visualization tasks

CHALLENGE 1 | JIGSAW CUT

For each puzzle, can you work out which of the dashed grid lines you should draw along in order to divide the given shape up into four identical regions? The regions may be rotated, but not reflected, relative to one another. You might find it helpful to copy out the shape first, since it may require some experimentation to find the solution.

> **To think laterally, challenge assumptions–don't fall back on accepted ways of thinking**

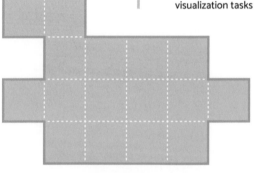

1 **EASY**

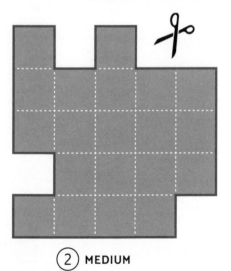

2 **MEDIUM**

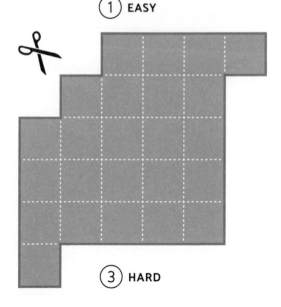

3 **HARD**

✦ Answers on p.186

CHALLENGE 2 | SNAKE

For each puzzle, shade some squares to form a single snake that starts and ends at the given squares. A snake is a path of adjacent squares that does not branch or cross over itself. The snake does not touch itself—not even diagonally, except when turning a corner. Numbers outside the grid specify the number of squares in their row or column that contain part of the snake.

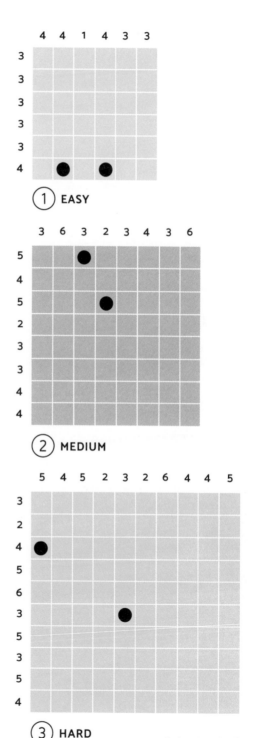

① **EASY**

② **MEDIUM**

③ **HARD**

✦ Answers on p.187

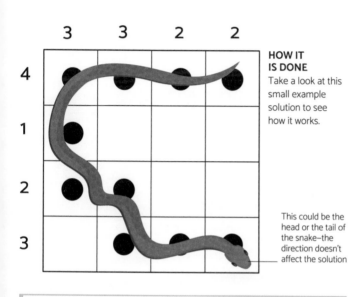

HOW IT IS DONE

Take a look at this small example solution to see how it works.

This could be the head or the tail of the snake—the direction doesn't affect the solution

TAKE IT FURTHER

Creative reasoning ability is valued by security agencies, some of which openly attract people who enjoy creating and solving puzzles. Puzzles are a great way to hone your creative thinking while having fun, and such skills help to keep the security industry ahead of threats such as cyber attacks. If you'd like to be a spy or to be involved in cybersecurity, you could start by working puzzles that demand lateral thinking and creative reasoning.

SPY

TRY MAKING MUSIC

Music is the most stimulating activity you can do for your brain. Nothing else gets as many parts of the brain working at the same time as playing or listening to music.

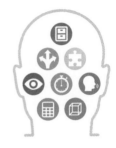

MAKING CONNECTIONS

Music is a multidisciplinary activity in the brain. There is no one center for processing music. Instead, areas associated with sound, sight, memory, motor skills, emotions, and decision-making all work together to interpret the stimuli coming from many parts of the body.

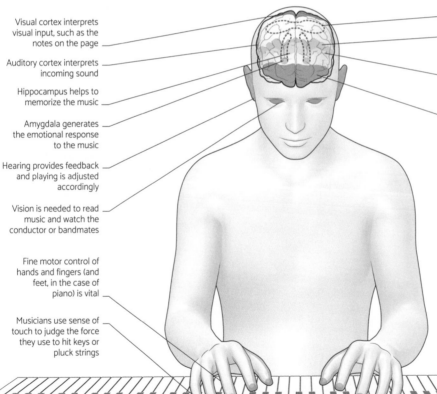

Visual cortex interprets visual input, such as the notes on the page

Auditory cortex interprets incoming sound

Hippocampus helps to memorize the music

Amygdala generates the emotional response to the music

Hearing provides feedback and playing is adjusted accordingly

Vision is needed to read music and watch the conductor or bandmates

Fine motor control of hands and fingers (and feet, in the case of piano) is vital

Musicians use sense of touch to judge the force they use to hit keys or pluck strings

Cerebellum marshals all the musician's movements

Somatosensory cortex interprets input from fingers and other parts making music

Motor cortex controls all the fine movements of the music-making body parts

Prefrontal cortex is needed for artistic interpretation

KEY

● Touch sensors and somatosensory cortex

● Eyes and visual cortex

● Ears and auditory cortex

● Fingers and motor cortex

● Prefrontal cortex

▪ ▪ ▪ Hippocampus

▪ ▪ ▪ Cerebellum

● Amygdala

EXERCISE 1 | BEAT IT

There is no music without rhythm, and "common notation," the most widely used system for writing music, tells you the rhythm using symbols for notes of different lengths. Notes are grouped into short periods of music called bars. In this exercise, there are four beats in a bar. These are counted as 1, 2, 3, 4; 1, 2, 3, 4, with an emphasis on each "1." See if you can use the information below to tap out these rhythms. You can clap, beat a drum, or tap the table. Count 1, 2, 3, 4 in each bar as you go, if it helps.

COUNT IT OUT

These symbols represent notes of different lengths. A whole note is the longest and is held for all four beats of a bar. A half note lasts two beats, a quarter one, an eighth is half a beat (you can count them "1-and-2-and..."). A sixteenth is a quarter beat (can be counted "1-e-and-a...").

WHOLE NOTE (FOUR BEATS)

HALF NOTE (TWO BEATS)

QUARTER NOTE (SINGLE BEAT)

EIGHTH NOTE (HALF BEAT)

SIXTEENTH NOTE (QUARTER BEAT)

Eighth and sixteenth notes have a tail (flag)

Four eighth notes linked with a beam

GROUPS OF SHORT NOTES

In musical notation, short notes are grouped for easy reading. Eighth notes are linked by a single beam, sixteenth notes by a double beam.

EXERCISE 2 | ... AND REST

For every beat in Exercise 1, there is an equivalent rest symbol that marks a place where no note is played. Rests are not pauses–you continue counting during the silence. Check the guide to rest symbols and the information on tied notes, below. Try to beat or clap the rhythms below. Remember not to sound rest notes and to hold over tied notes for their combined length.

REST SYMBOLS

Resting beats have their own set of symbols that correspond to the notes of different lengths in the first exercise. For example, a quarter rest is the silent equivalent of a quarter beat.

There are 16 of these in a 4/4 bar

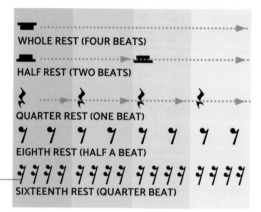

WHOLE REST (FOUR BEATS)

HALF REST (TWO BEATS)

QUARTER REST (ONE BEAT)

EIGHTH REST (HALF A BEAT)

SIXTEENTH REST (QUARTER BEAT)

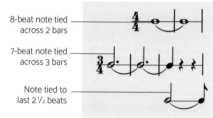

8-beat note tied across 2 bars

7-beat note tied across 3 bars

Note tied to last 2½ beats

WHEN ONE SYMBOL IS NOT ENOUGH

A curved line, or tie, between notes tells you to hold the note for the combined length of the tied notes, either because the intended sound crosses between bars, or it lasts for an irregular number of beats that doesn't have its own symbol.

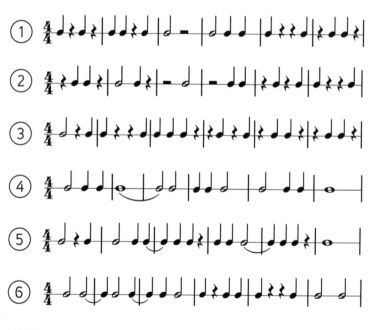

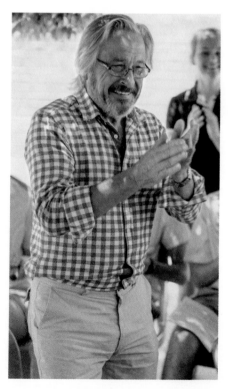

JOIN IN

The rhythm of a piece of music can be infectious. Those not playing can join in by clapping or tapping their feet in time to the beat. You may not even be aware you're doing it!

EXERCISE 3 | DOTTED RHYTHMS

Another way of showing that a note should be held for longer is the dotted note and its corresponding rest. Dotted note and rest values are half as long again as their undotted versions. A dotted quarter is played for 1½ beats, rather than just one beat. Try beating out these dotted rhythms.

DOTTED NOTES
Dots save having to put in extra notes and tie them together. A dotted half note (top) is equal to three beats–two for the half and one for a quarter.

DOTTED RESTS
Dotted rests work the same way. A dotted eighth rest (top) is the same as an eighth rest plus a sixteenth rest (three quarter beats). A dotted quarter rest (bottom) lasts three half beats.

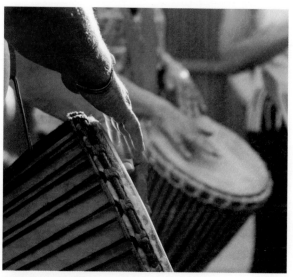

BEAT OF THE DRUM
Most types of music rely on a strong percussive beat. Fast beats raise the heart rate of listeners, prompting a sense of urgency and excitement. Slower beats have a calming effect and can relieve tension.

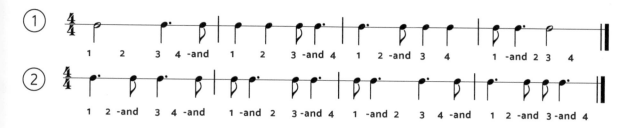

EXERCISE 4 | NOW BOTH HANDS

Can you tap one rhythm with one hand and another rhythm with the other? It's harder than you think. Using a hand drum, or just the table top, tap the top line with your right hand and the bottom line with your left hand. Try each hand separately until you get the feel of both rhythms, then put them together.

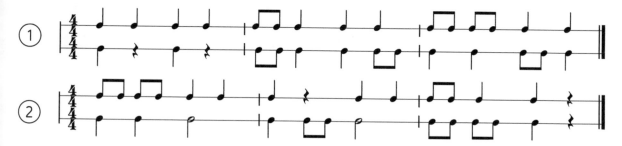

EXERCISE 5 | **TIME SIGNATURES**

At the start of any piece of music is the time signature. This tells you how many beats are in a bar of music. The signature 4/4 tells you there are four beats, while 3/4 has three beats and 2/4 has two. The number of beats controls the rhythm of the piece– a typical marching rhythm is 4/4, while 3/4 can be a waltz. 5/4 is a rarer time signature, giving an odd, lilting rhythm. Try tapping out these examples.

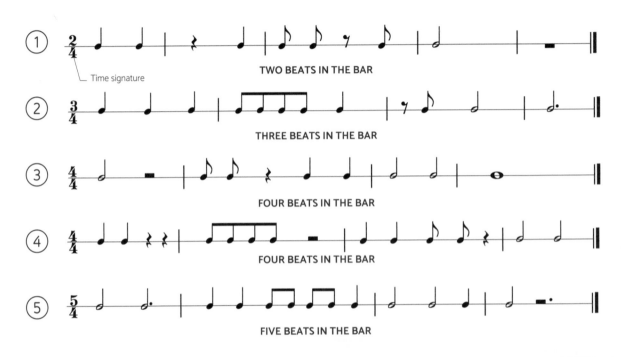

① TWO BEATS IN THE BAR

Time signature

② THREE BEATS IN THE BAR

③ FOUR BEATS IN THE BAR

④ FOUR BEATS IN THE BAR

⑤ FIVE BEATS IN THE BAR

TAKE IT FURTHER

Music is so varied that there is something for everyone. Whether listening to it or joining in, you can find genres that can lift or soothe your mood. Try something new occasionally to expand your repertoire and keep your brain challenged.

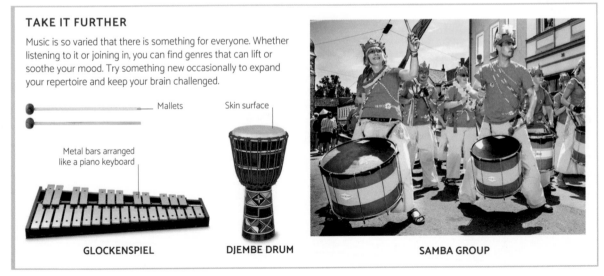

Mallets

Metal bars arranged like a piano keyboard

Skin surface

GLOCKENSPIEL

DJEMBE DRUM

SAMBA GROUP

EXERCISE 6 | PITCH PERFECT

So far, we have looked only at rhythm, but to add melody, you need notes of different pitches. To show pitch, music is written on a staff (or stave)–a series of five lines. The notes, named with the letters A–G, sit on the lines or in the spaces of the staff. The clef symbol, right at the beginning, tells you which positions represent which notes. For high notes, the treble clef is used, while the bass clef is used for lower notes. Using this information, can you name the notes on the staffs below?

READING THE STAFF

Notes are centered on either a line or a space on the staff. If a note is too high or low to fit on the staff, it sits on a short "ledger line." The C on the first ledger line of the bass-clef staff is the same C as that on the first ledger line at the bottom of the treble-clef staff.

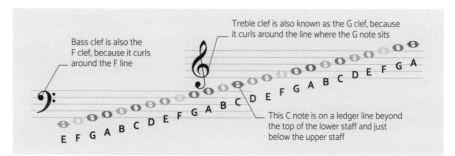

Bass clef is also the F clef, because it curls around the F line

Treble clef is also known as the G clef, because it curls around the line where the G note sits

This C note is on a ledger line beyond the top of the lower staff and just below the upper staff

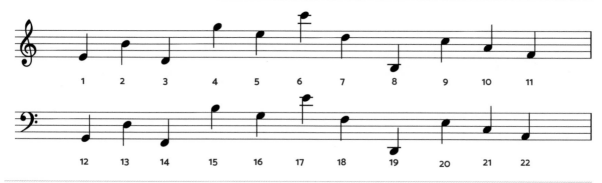

EXERCISE 7 | SHARPS AND FLATS

The sequence of notes C D E F G A B C forms a scale that sounds natural and pleasing, but the pitches of these notes are not evenly spaced. Some are spaced by whole tones, others by half this, or a semitone. To name all the notes, including those between the whole tones, we need sharp and flat symbols. A sharp raises the note by a semitone, a flat symbol lowers it by a semitone. Can you name the notes below?

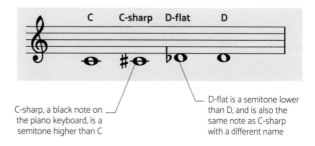

C-sharp, a black note on the piano keyboard, is a semitone higher than C

D-flat is a semitone lower than D, and is also the same note as C-sharp with a different name

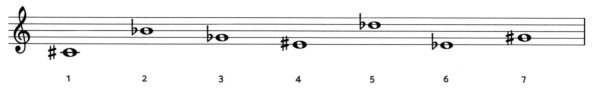

TRY PIANO

The piano is a great challenge to the brain, requiring some areas of the brain to work on multiple things at the same time: hands, feet, eyes, ears, and spatial awareness.

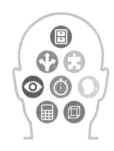

THINKING SKILLS

Coordinates movements in limbs and body

•

Activates visual, sound, and motor cortices

•

Reinforces memory and hard-wires repeated actions

EXERCISE 1 | **LEARN THE KEYBOARD**

A piano is a large and expensive instrument, but it possesses a range and versatility other instruments don't have. If you don't have room for a piano, try an electronic keyboard, or even a piano app for your phone or tablet. It may not have the same range, but it's enough to get you started.

NOTES AND KEYS

Piano music is written on a pair of staffs, one for each hand. The piano keys play notes written on the lines and spaces of the staff.

The vertical position of each note tells you the pitch

Treble clef tells you these are the high notes, played with the right hand

Bass clef tells you these are the low notes, normally played with the left hand

STAFF

Left hand Right Hand

C D E F G A B C D E F G A B C D E F G A B C D E F G A B C

KEYBOARD

A lower C, one octave lower than middle C

Middle C

A high C, two octaves higher than middle C

① **WHITE NOTES**
Locate middle C, which is a white key found just to the left of two black keys near the center of the keyboard (or the lock, if it has one). Play all the white notes to the right in turn, until you get to the next C. An interval of eight notes is called an octave. Now with the left hand, play all the white notes to the left of middle C until you hit the C an octave below.

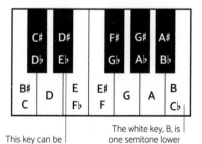

This key can be either D-sharp or E-flat

The white key, B, is one semitone lower than C and can be called C-flat

② **BLACK NOTES**
Now play the black notes. Depending on the musical context, the black keys can be seen as sharps (♯)—a semitone higher than the white key to the left, or flats (♭)—a semitone lower than the white key to the right. However, not all sharps and flats are black notes—in some contexts, the white notes have sharp or flat names, too.

EXERCISE 2 | PLAY SCALES

Learning to play scales allows you to move around a keyboard fluently and easily. It helps you to develop a spatial awareness of the keys in both hands and the relationships between the notes. Play first with the right hand and then with the left. Then try both together. Aim for a smooth, even movement. Playing scales requires you to read two staffs of music at once. Start with the easy scale of C Major (this has no sharps or flats), then try the other scales, which have increasing numbers of black notes.

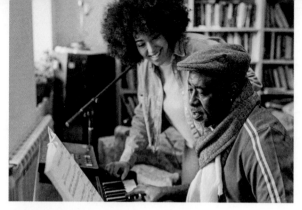

FIND A TEACHER

You can only learn so much on your own. A teacher or experienced player can advise on technique and improve your skills in reading music.

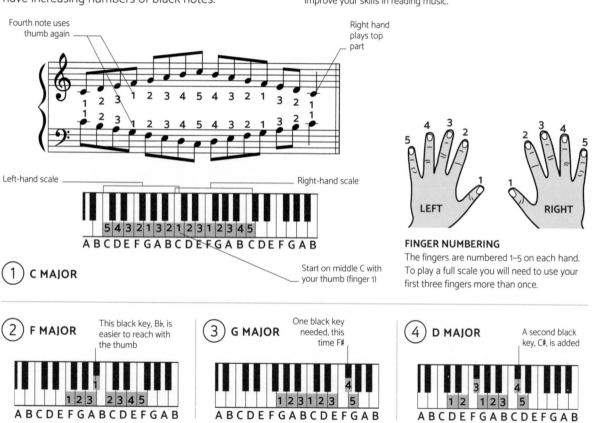

Fourth note uses thumb again

Right hand plays top part

Left-hand scale

Right-hand scale

1 2 3 1 2 3 4 5 4 3 2 1 3 2 1

5 4 3 2 1 3 2 1 2 3 1 2 3 4 5

A B C D E F G A B C D E F G A B C D E F G A B

1 C MAJOR

Start on middle C with your thumb (finger 1)

FINGER NUMBERING

The fingers are numbered 1–5 on each hand. To play a full scale you will need to use your first three fingers more than once.

LEFT   RIGHT

---

2 F MAJOR

This black key, B♭, is easier to reach with the thumb

1 2 3   2 3 4 5

A B C D E F G A B C D E F G A B

3 G MAJOR

One black key needed, this time F♯

1 2 3 1 2 3   5

A B C D E F G A B C D E F G A B

4 D MAJOR

A second black key, C♯, is added

1 2   1 2 3   5

A B C D E F G A B C D E F G A B

5 A MAJOR

G♯ makes it three black keys

1 2   1 2   3   3 4   5

A B C D E F G A B C D E F G A B

6 E MAJOR

D♯ is the fourth black key

1   1 2   2 3   3 4   5

A B C D E F G A B C D E F G A B

7 B MAJOR

B major uses all five black keys

1   1   2 3   2 3 4   5

A B C D E F G A B C D E F G A B

EXERCISE 3 | STRIKE A CHORD

Chords consist of multiple notes played together and are common in piano music, especially in the left hand, supporting the melody. Try playing these chords. Listen, and you may hear that they are three versions of the same chord—C Major.

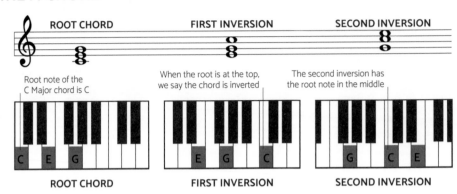

ROOT CHORD   FIRST INVERSION   SECOND INVERSION

Root note of the C Major chord is C

When the root is at the top, we say the chord is inverted

The second inversion has the root note in the middle

ROOT CHORD   FIRST INVERSION   SECOND INVERSION

EXERCISE 4 | A CHANGE OF MOOD

Notes may be added or substituted in a major chord to give the chord a different tone or mood. This is usually done by flattening or sharpening (altering by a semitone) one or more of the notes in the chord.

(1) This is how some common chords look in the key of "C." Play them and listen to the difference in sound. Major chords sound bright and happy, while minor chords are sad and subdued. Diminished chords have a tense quality, whereas augmented chords have a sense of suspense and expectancy.

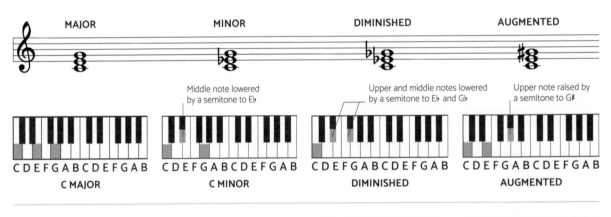

MAJOR   MINOR   DIMINISHED   AUGMENTED

Middle note lowered by a semitone to E♭

Upper and middle notes lowered by a semitone to E♭ and G♭

Upper note raised by a semitone to G♯

C D E F G A B C D E F G A B — C MAJOR
C D E F G A B C D E F G A B — C MINOR
C D E F G A B C D E F G A B — DIMINISHED
C D E F G A B C D E F G A B — AUGMENTED

(2) Experiment to see if you can find major, minor, diminished, and augmented chords in these different keys. Lower the third note a semitone to make a minor, or raise the fifth note to augment it. When you start on a different keynote, as in the scales, the pattern of black notes changes, adding to the challenge. Start with these major chords.

To make a minor chord out of E Major, lower this G♯ a semitone down to G

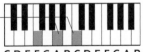

C D E F G A B C D E F G A B — E MAJOR

C D E F G A B C D E F G A B — D MAJOR

To make a diminished F chord, lower the A to A♭ and the C to C♭ (usually known as B)

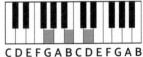

C D E F G A B C D E F G A B — F MAJOR

C D E F G A B C D E F G A B — G MAJOR

EXERCISE 5 | CHORDS IN C MAJOR

Every scale produces seven different chords. These are the chords for C Major. Three of the chords are major and four are minor (m). Chords are numbered using Roman numerals: uppercase for major chords, lowercase for minor chords. Play them all and listen to how they sound. Like guitar chords (see pp.112–15), they can provide backing to songs.

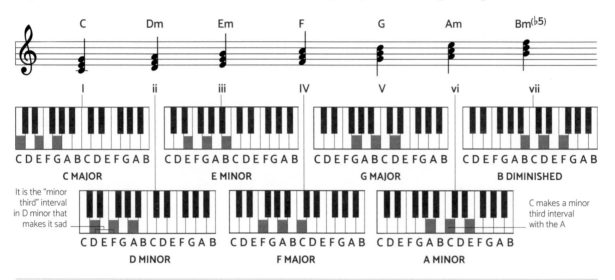

| C | Dm | Em | F | G | Am | Bm(♭5) |
| I | ii | iii | IV | V | vi | vii |

C D E F G A B C D E F G A B
C MAJOR

C D E F G A B C D E F G A B
E MINOR

C D E F G A B C D E F G A B
G MAJOR

C D E F G A B C D E F G A B
B DIMINISHED

It is the "minor third" interval in D minor that makes it sad

C D E F G A B C D E F G A B
D MINOR

C D E F G A B C D E F G A B
F MAJOR

C D E F G A B C D E F G A B
A MINOR

C makes a minor third interval with the A

EXERCISE 6 | CHORD PROGRESSION

Chords move, or progress, with the melody. One of the most common progressions, used in all types of music, is the I–V–vi–IV sequence. Play the sequence below and see whether you can relate it to a song you know, such as "Let it Be" by the Beatles, or Bob Marley's "No Woman, No Cry." Then see if you can figure out how the chords progress through the rest of the song. Check the keyboards above if you need a reminder of which keys to play.

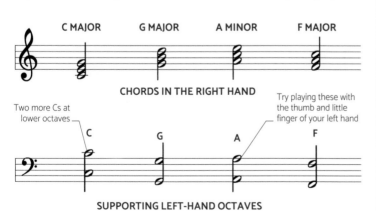

| C MAJOR | G MAJOR | A MINOR | F MAJOR |

CHORDS IN THE RIGHT HAND

Two more Cs at lower octaves

Try playing these with the thumb and little finger of your left hand

C G A F

SUPPORTING LEFT-HAND OCTAVES

TAKE IT FURTHER

The key to learning any instrument is practice. Take it slowly at first and set yourself a daily goal, such as playing a scale fluently. Practice sight-reading a new piece once a week. This will help with fingering and your knowledge of musical notation.

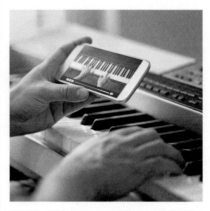

PIANO APPS CAN HELP WITH TECHNIQUE

TRY GUITAR

You can carry a guitar to produce music anywhere. It can play chords as well as melodies, so it sounds good unaccompanied or in a group. Guitar is a great introduction to making music.

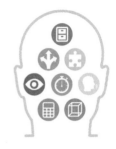

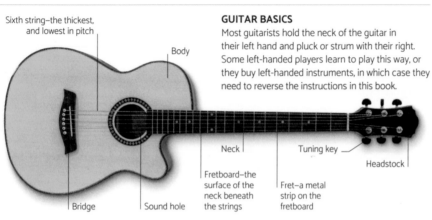

Sixth string–the thickest, and lowest in pitch

Body

Neck

Tuning key

Headstock

Fretboard–the surface of the neck beneath the strings

Fret–a metal strip on the fretboard

Bridge

Sound hole

GUITAR BASICS

Most guitarists hold the neck of the guitar in their left hand and pluck or strum with their right. Some left-handed players learn to play this way, or they buy left-handed instruments, in which case they need to reverse the instructions in this book.

THINKING SKILLS

Develops fine motor skills

•

Stimulates the senses

•

Activates nearly every part of the brain, including parts resposible for movement, memory, and emotion

EXERCISE 1 | TUNE IT UP

Strings slacken with time, and this sends the notes off-key. Each time you pick up the guitar, check it's in tune. Tuning it by ear is a good mental exercise, although an electric tuner makes it easier. The strings are tuned to the notes E–A–D–G–B–E.

(1) The sixth string should be tuned to a low E. Check the pitch with an electric tuner, piano, or a piano app on your phone. Listen while turning the peg until the string's pitch matches the reference pitch.

(2) Now use the sixth string to tune the fifth. Press the sixth string down on the fifth fret to play an A. Keep your finger on the fret and play the open (unfretted) fifth string. Turn the peg on the fifth string until its pitch matches the sixth string's.

(3) Now use the fifth string to tune the fourth. Press the fifth string down on the fifth fret to sound a D. Tune the fourth string until it matches.

(4) Now tune the third string to a G by pressing on the fifth fret of the fourth string.

(5) Tune the second string by pressing on the fourth fret of the third string to sound a B.

(6) Finally, tune the first string to a high E by pressing on the fifth fret of the second string.

(7) Check the tuning by sounding consecutive pairs of strings from sixth to first–they might need more tweaking. Play a few chords and strum across all the strings.

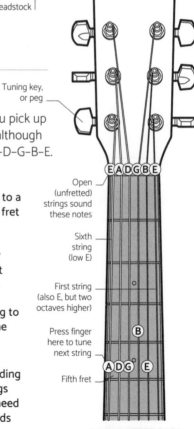

Tuning key, or peg

Open (unfretted) strings sound these notes

Sixth string (low E)

First string (also E, but two octaves higher)

Press finger here to tune next string

Fifth fret

GUITAR FRETBOARD

EXERCISE 2 | THREE-STRING CHORDS

Playing a guitar chord requires you to sound the strings almost simultaneously. You can play chords with just the three high strings, which makes it easier to start learning them. If you hear a "buzz" as you play the chord, one or more fingers is not in the right place or not applying the right pressure. Adjust your fingers until it goes.

① **STRUM DOWN**
Using your thumb or a pick, strum with a firm, even stroke, moving from the wrist, not the arm.

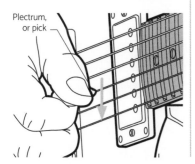

Plectrum, or pick

② **RECOVER POSITION**
After the down-stroke, return the pick to the start. You can also strum upward, reversing this pattern.

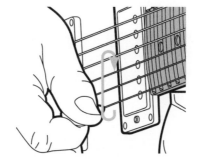

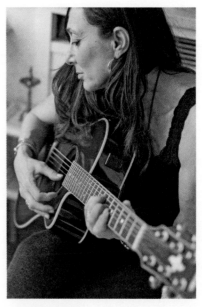

MAKING MUSIC
Your first chords can be played by strumming the higher three strings with your thumb—or with a plectrum, or pick.

③ **C MAJOR**
To play C major (or simply "C") with three strings, you need just one finger. Keep your thumb behind the neck, providing light resistance to the finger pressure.

Open third string plays G (the fifth note of C major)

Press on the second string with your first finger to play C, the root note

Open first string plays E (the major third note of C)

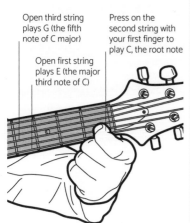

④ **MOVE FROM C TO G**
To achieve your first chord transition, lift your first finger, and in the same moment, plant your third finger on the third fret, on the first string.

Third finger moves to third fret on the first string

First finger releases pressure on second string

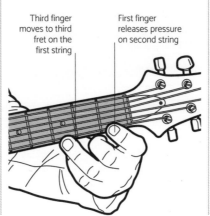

⑤ **G MAJOR**
This chord is made from the the open third and second strings (these play G and B respectively), and the first string, raised to a higher G by your finger on the third fret.

Third finger raises the pitch of the first string to a high G

Take care not to mute the 2nd string

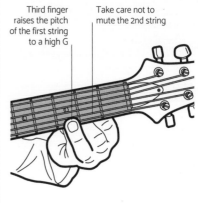

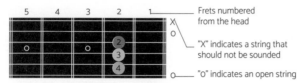

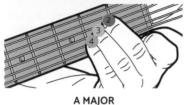

Frets numbered from the head

"X" indicates a string that should not be sounded

"o" indicates an open string

A MAJOR

TABS
Guitar chord fingering can be pictured with diagrams called tabs (tabulation), such as the one above for A major.

EXERCISE 3 | CHORD PROGRESSIONS

Many songs are backed by sequences of chords called progressions. The most common follows the pattern I–IV–V. In the key of C, these chords would be C, F, and G—the first, fourth, and fifth chords of the scale (see p.111). Learn these three chords, and you can play a song in C. If you learn D major, you can play a I–IV–V song in the key of G (using G, C, and D chords). A minor chord or two gives you the option of songs with the I–V–vi–IV pattern (see p.111). With confidence and practice, you can bring in four, five, or six strings.

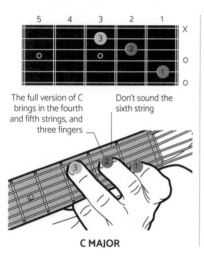

The full version of C brings in the fourth and fifth strings, and three fingers

Don't sound the sixth string

C MAJOR

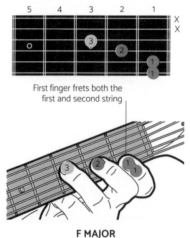

First finger frets both the first and second string

F MAJOR

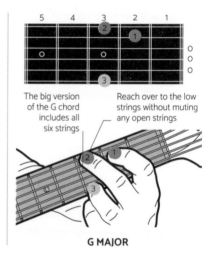

The big version of the G chord includes all six strings

Reach over to the low strings without muting any open strings

G MAJOR

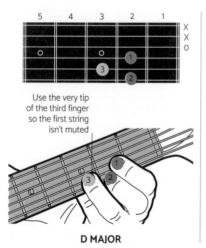

Use the very tip of the third finger so the first string isn't muted

D MAJOR

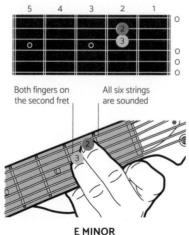

Both fingers on the second fret

All six strings are sounded

E MINOR

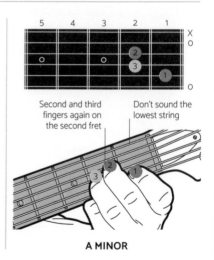

Second and third fingers again on the second fret

Don't sound the lowest string

A MINOR

EXERCISE 4 | PICKING

Guitar is not just about playing chords. Riffs, solos, and other melodic playing requires picking of single strings. To play melody, you need to learn the position of notes on the fretboard and practice playing scales.

① USING A PICK, OR PLECTRUM

Lightly rest your palm on the bridge, keeping your unused fingers loosely tucked in. Angle the pick for lighter strokes.

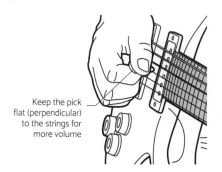

Keep the pick flat (perpendicular) to the strings for more volume

② FINGER PICKING

Keep your hand floating without resting on the body or bridge. Long nails are an advantage on steel strings and necessary on nylon-strung guitars.

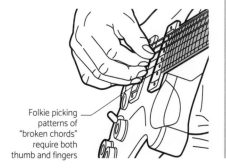

Folkie picking patterns of "broken chords" require both thumb and fingers

TAKE IT FURTHER

Once you have mastered the chords demonstrated by the tabs and illustrations on these pages, there are hundreds more to explore, and several ways of playing the same chord.

- Find a more experienced player who can give you tips and advice.

- Learn the shortcut fingerings for chords, which can make it easier to play progressions.

- If six strings are too many to cope with, try a ukulele, which has only four.

Sixth string

This is an electric guitar fretboard, with 22 frets

From one fret to the next is one semitone–from a white to an adjacent black note on the piano keyboard

Fret positions with sharps and flats have two names, but they are the same note

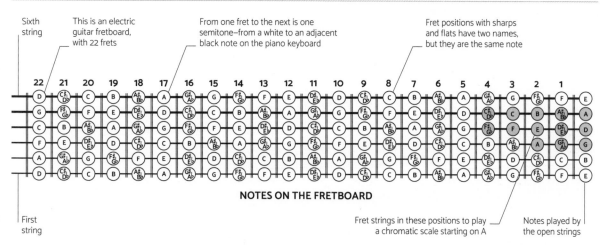

NOTES ON THE FRETBOARD

First string

Fret strings in these positions to play a chromatic scale starting on A

Notes played by the open strings

③ UP AND DOWN

It's easy to remember that you play sharps going up the neck and flats as you go down. Try playing all the notes on a string in both directions.

④ NEXT STRING

Move on to the next string. Practice for 15–30 minutes a day until you can immediately sound a note on a given string without looking.

⑤ SCALES

Learn to play a scale using different strings to save moving so far on the fretboard. A suggested pattern is highlighted in yellow above.

⑥ SHORT BURSTS

When you start playing, it will hurt both your finger pads and muscles. Practice in short bursts, and eventually your fingers will toughen up.

TRY DRAWING

As we grow up, our brains learn to edit out a lot of what we see, focusing only on what is important. Drawing forces us to look at things differently, since it relies on close observation. It is also good for relieving stress and improving memory.

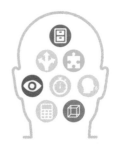

EXERCISE 1 | GET THE PROPORTIONS RIGHT

For a drawing to be realistic, the objects depicted need to be a recognizable shape and the right size in relation to each other. You can measure the height and width of one object compared with another by using a pencil held out in front of you with a straight arm. This simple measuring technique, known as sighting, is also useful for checking the distance between objects.

① Align the top of your pencil with the top of the line you are measuring. Close one eye and move your thumb up and down the pencil until it matches the length of the line.

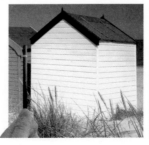

② Keeping your thumb in place, transfer the pencil to the page, holding it against the correct line of your drawing. Adjust the length of the line you have drawn to match.

Check your line is the right length

EXERCISE 2 | SEEING SHAPES

Most objects and scenes can be broken down into simple geometric shapes, such as squares, circles, or ovals (like this cup and saucer). Doing this will help you to observe things more accurately. First, draw the overall shapes you can see, then break the object down into smaller shapes before adding detail.

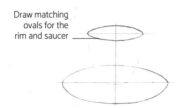

Draw matching ovals for the rim and saucer

① Draw lines to mark the center of the cup rim and the saucer. Measure their height and depth (see Exercise 1), then draw two ovals.

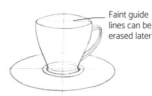

Faint guide lines can be erased later

② Now draw two smaller ovals on the saucer where the cup rests. Study the cup, then sketch its sloping sides, handle, and curved base.

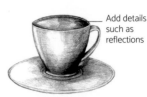

Add details such as reflections

③ Once you have sketched an accurate outline, you can add detail and shading, giving the cup and saucer a three-dimensional form.

EXERCISE 3 |
DRAWING PEOPLE

You can simplify the human form in exactly the same way as objects. Start by measuring the proportions with a pencil and figure out the scale so you can fit the whole figure on the paper. The head is a useful unit of measuring. Use it to figure out the relative sizes of the limbs and torso.

Use the head to get the proportions right—an average adult stands at 7–8 heads tall

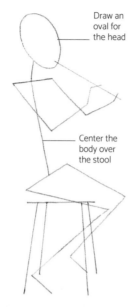

Draw an oval for the head

Center the body over the stool

(1) Use simple lines (a stick figure) to plot how the basic shapes relate to each other and position the body on the stool.

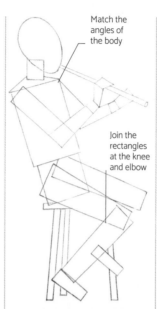

Match the angles of the body

Join the rectangles at the knee and elbow

(2) Divide the body into geometric shapes: a triangle for the shoulders, a rectangular torso, and rectangles for the limbs.

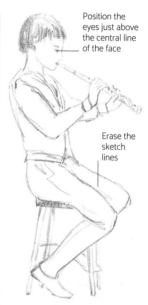

Position the eyes just above the central line of the face

Erase the sketch lines

(3) Now refine the figure, modifying the shapes according to what you see. Erase the old sketch marks once you have done this.

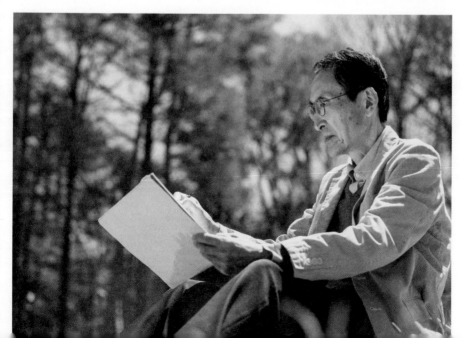

DRAW ANYWHERE
Carrying a sketchbook around allows you to draw when and what you want. You can record your thoughts, doodle, or try out different compositions. You can also exercise your memory by committing a scene to paper once you have moved away.

EXERCISE 4 | DRAW A PORTRAIT

Faces are one of the most interesting subjects to draw, because they look different from every angle, and a person's expression changes from one moment to the next. You can draw a portrait from life or a photograph. Alternatively, you can draw a self-portrait using a mirror–you'll see yourself in a whole new light! Use a charcoal pencil for this exercise.

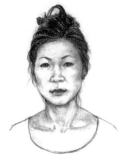

CHARCOAL PORTRAIT

(1) Holding the pencil loosely, draw the simple shapes of the head. Mark the eyebrows, eyes, tip of the nose, and mouth.

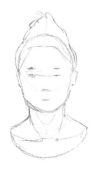

(2) Look to see where shadows fall on the face, then block in these shapes. Use an eraser to blend and highlight areas.

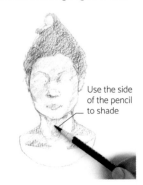

Use the side of the pencil to shade

EXERCISE 5 | PERSPECTIVE

Perspective is about placing objects within the space you are drawing. Understanding how it works will help you to re-create depth and space. All parallel lines appear to meet at the same point on the horizon–the vanishing point. Knowing this enables you to draw objects in proportion. Separating a scene into three planes – background, middle ground, and foreground – can also give an impression of depth and distance.

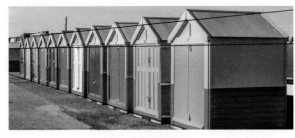

LINEAR PERSPECTIVE

Vanishing point

Lines converge with distance

Closer huts appear bigger

(1) To find the vanishing point, draw lines along the tops and bases of the beach huts. The lines will eventually meet.

(2) Transfer the lines of perspective to your paper and use them to size the beach huts correctly relative to one another.

(1) **BACKGROUND** In the far background of a scene, objects appear paler and less distinct. You can exaggerate this effect to imply greater distance.

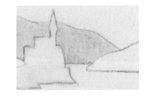

(2) **MIDDLE GROUND** Objects in the middle ground appear sharper than those in the background. Try overlapping elements to make the contrast more obvious.

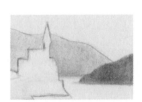

(3) **FOREGROUND** You can see objects in the foreground more clearly than those behind them. Add detail and tonal contrast to create an impression of depth.

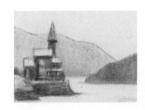

3 Now set the features in the face, working down from the eyebrows. Draw the iris of each eye before you do the pupils.

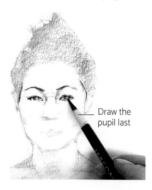

Draw the pupil last

4 Note the distance between the eyes and nostrils before drawing the nose. For the lips, work from the center line outward.

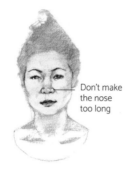

Don't make the nose too long

5 Now go back over the shape of the face, from chin to jawline to ears. Build up marks in the direction of hair growth.

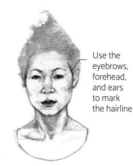

Use the eyebrows, forehead, and ears to mark the hairline

TAKE IT FURTHER

Drawing is a popular pastime among older people, and it's a good way to get out and about. You can join a local art class, where you'll meet like-minded people and hone your skills. There are lots of different media you can experiment with, too.

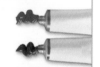

WATERCOLORS

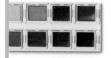

OIL PAINTS

CHALK

CRAYON

PEN

CHARCOAL PENCIL

COLORED PENCIL

EXERCISE 6 | SCALE UP A COMPOSITION

To draw a picture on a larger or smaller scale than the original, set out a grid over the original image on tracing paper. Transfer the grid to your paper, keeping the proportions the same. The grid helps you to see which elements should be in which square, so you can reproduce the image accurately.

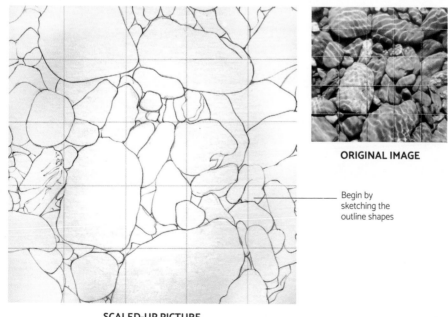

ORIGINAL IMAGE

Begin by sketching the outline shapes

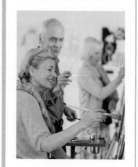

PAINTING CLASS

SCALED-UP PICTURE

TRY CHESS

Chess is a game of strategy in which the goal is to trap your opponent's king so that it has no escape, which is called checkmate. To achieve this, you need to know the different pieces and how they can move around the board.

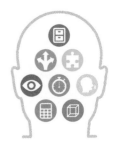

THINKING SKIILS

Improves planning and strategic thinking

•

Enhances problem-solving

•

Improves concentration

CHESSBOARD

A chessboard is made up of an 8x8 grid of 64 squares, alternating between black and white. Each player starts with 16 pieces. If a piece lands on an occupied square, that piece is captured and removed from the board.

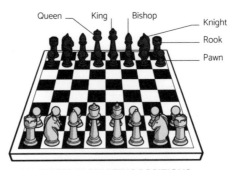

Queen — King — Bishop — Knight — Rook — Pawn

ALL PIECES IN STARTING POSITIONS

CHALLENGE 1 | **PAWN**

For their first move, pawns can move two squares, but only one square after that. To capture another piece they must move one square diagonally. If a pawn reaches the other end of the board, it can be changed into any other piece.

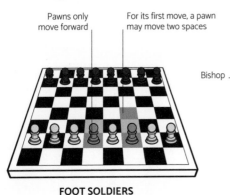

Pawns only move forward

For its first move, a pawn may move two spaces

FOOT SOLDIERS

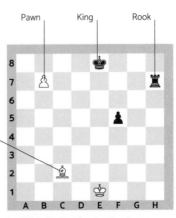

Pawn — King — Rook

Bishop

In this challenge, both players have three pieces left, but it is white's turn. What is the best move for white in the situation shown here?

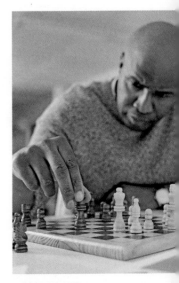

DON'T TOUCH
Plan your move mentally before taking action. Once you touch one of your pieces during your turn, you have to move that piece. When you remove your hand, your turn is over.

✦ Answers on p.187

CHALLENGE 2 | BISHOP

Bishops move diagonally backward or forward across any number of empty squares. A bishop must always stay on the same color squares it started on.

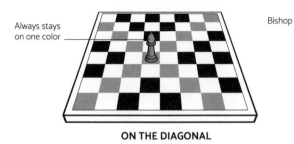

Always stays on one color

ON THE DIAGONAL

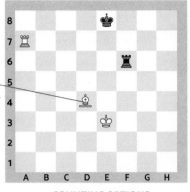

Bishop

How many squares, in total, can the bishop move to on the board shown here? And which piece can the white bishop capture?

COUNTING OPTIONS

CHALLENGE 3 | KNIGHT

Knights move in a capital-L shape. This can either be two squares forward or backward and one sideways, or one square forward or backward and two sideways.

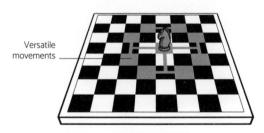

Versatile movements

KNIGHT MOVES

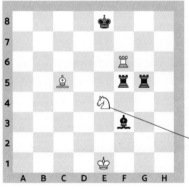

Knight

A knight may jump over other pieces without capturing them. Which piece on this board is vulnerable to the knight? Remember, you cannot capture your own pieces.

LEAP INTO ACTION

CHALLENGE 4 | ROOK

Also sometimes called a castle, a rook can move forward, backward, or sideways in a straight line along any number of empty squares.

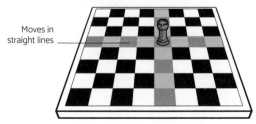

Moves in straight lines

MOVEABLE FORTRESS

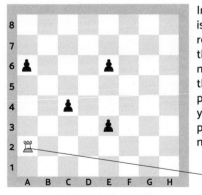

Rook

In this example it is possible for the rook to capture all the pawns in five moves. Assume that none of the pawns move. Can you take all four pawns in just five moves?

PICKING OFF PAWNS

✦ Answers on p.187

CHALLENGE 5 | QUEEN

The most useful piece on the board, the queen can move in any straight direction, including diagonally, over any number of squares. It cannot jump over pieces but can stop before them or capture them.

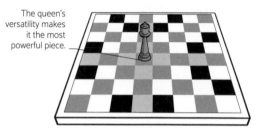

The queen's versatility makes it the most powerful piece.

THE MOST POWERFUL PIECE

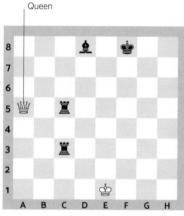

Queen

The strength of the queen also makes it a piece to target and care should be taken when deciding where to attack. Which piece can the queen safely capture here?

DO NOT SACRIFICE THE QUEEN

CHALLENGE 6 | KING

The king can move one square in any direction. The object of the game is to capture your opponent's king. When your king is in a position to be taken, it is in check. There are three ways to avoid check: capture the checking piece; block the move; or move your king out of the way. If the king is in check and there is no escape, it is called checkmate and the game is over.

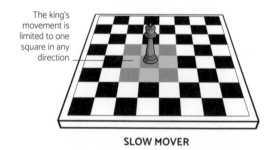

The king's movement is limited to one square in any direction

SLOW MOVER

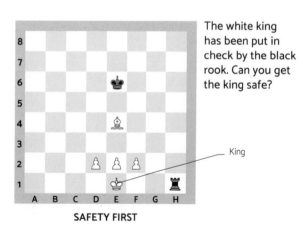

King

The white king has been put in check by the black rook. Can you get the king safe?

SAFETY FIRST

In this situation, the white king is in check. Can you find a move that gets the king safe?

King

PLANNING AN ESCAPE

✦ Answers on p.187

CHALLENGE 7 | **ACHIEVING CHECKMATE**

To win a game of chess requires strategy, as you need to protect your own king, while also trying to trap your opponent's king in checkmate. To achieve checkmate often requires more than one piece to ensure your opponent cannot prevent the move or escape.

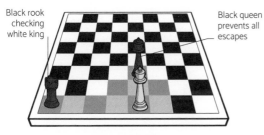

Black rook checking white king

Black queen prevents all escapes

OUT OF MOVES

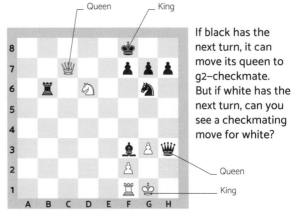

Queen

King

If black has the next turn, it can move its queen to g2–checkmate. But if white has the next turn, can you see a checkmating move for white?

Queen

King

QUICK VICTORY, OR DEFEAT

✦Answer on p.187

TAKE IT FURTHER

Find someone who plays chess to give you a game or join a chess club. You can also try solving chess challenges in magazines and newspapers or download a digital chess game or app and pit your wits against chess-playing AI. Alternatively, try other strategy board games, such as Mahjong, Backgammon,

Go, or Hive. Mahjong uses a set of 144 tiles and it is usually played by four people, although there are three-player versions. Backgammon is one of the oldest board games and uses two dice, which makes it a game of skill and luck. Pieces are moved along the board and the first player to clear all their pieces wins.

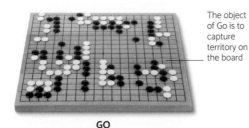

The object of Go is to capture territory on the board

GO

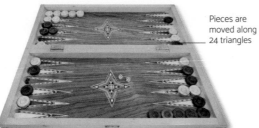

Pieces are moved along 24 triangles

BACKGAMMON

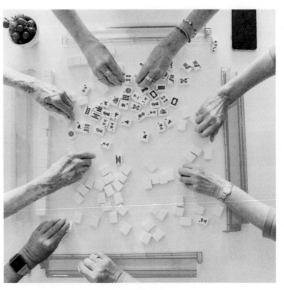

MAHJONG

TRY BRIDGE

Bridge is a great way to exercise your brain while being sociable. Each game brings a unique set of problems and solutions, and your planning, counting, and reasoning skills will be put to the test.

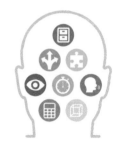

THINKING SKILLS

Boosts memory

•

Enhances problem-solving and number skills

•

Improves concentration

•

Requires quick thinking

EXERCISE 1 | GET STARTED

All you need to play bridge is a deck of 52 cards, a table, and two opposing pairs of players (North/South and East/West). The object of the game is to win tricks for your side (out of a total of 13). A trick is made up of four cards, one from each player.

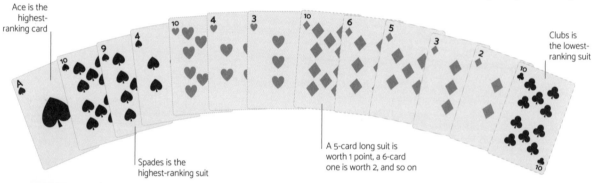

Ace is the highest-ranking card

Spades is the highest-ranking suit

A 5-card long suit is worth 1 point, a 6-card one is worth 2, and so on

Clubs is the lowest-ranking suit

① SORT YOUR CARDS
One player starts as the dealer and deals 13 cards (a hand) to all four players. Each player then arranges their hand by suit (spades, hearts, diamonds, and clubs) and rank (Ace, King, Queen, Jack, and so on).

② VALUE YOUR HAND
The next stage is to value your hand. You can get an idea of what it is worth by adding up high-card points (4 points for an Ace, 3 for a King, 2 for a Queen, and 1 for a Jack) and long suits (five or more cards from one suit).

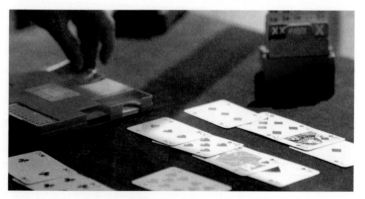

FAIR PLAY
In bridge, you are not allowed to use any secret signals to give your partner information about your hand. Don't say more than you need to when bidding, and use the same tone of voice throughout.

Bridge is the world's most popular partnership card game

EXERCISE 2 | BIDDING

Bidding is a way of communicating the strengths and weaknesses of your hand to your partner before play begins. A bid consists of a number, from 1 to 7, and a suit or "no trump" (NT). Having valued their hand, each player must bid for the minimum number of tricks they think they can win (six plus the number given in the bid). If a player has lots of cards from one suit, they may bid to make that the trump suit (which outranks other suits). If their hand is evenly distributed, they may bid for no trumps. Players can choose to bid or "pass."

① The dealer opens the bidding, and bidding moves clockwise. The hierarchy of suits (NT, ♠, ♥, ♦, ♣) determines the bidding. If 1♥ is the opening bid, the next hand must pass or make a higher bid (at least 1♠).

② The bidding continues around the table, until three players in a row pass. The last bid wins the auction. Here, the North/South pair has bid 5♥, so their target, or contract, is to win 11 tricks (6+5) with hearts as trumps.

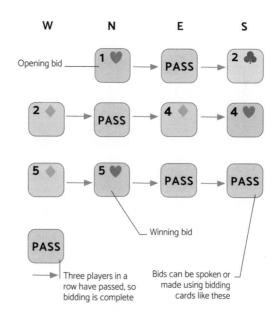

N

W   The dealer (North) makes the first bid

E

East will be next to bid

S

W   N   E   S

Opening bid → 1♥ → PASS → 2♣

2♦ → PASS → 4♦ → 4♥

5♦ → 5♥ → PASS → PASS

PASS

Three players in a row have passed, so bidding is complete

Winning bid

Bids can be spoken or made using bidding cards like these

BIDDING IN MINIBRIDGE

Minibridge is often used to introduce children to bridge because it has a simpler bidding system. First, each player calculates their hand by adding up their high-card points. The dealer announces their points, followed, in a clockwise direction, by the other players. The total should add up to 40. The player with the most points becomes the declarer, and their partner becomes the dummy (see Exercise 3). If both pairs have 20 points, the cards are redealt. Next, with the dummy's hand faceup on the table, the declarer chooses a contract: "part-score" (a goal of 7 tricks) or "game" (a goal of 9 tricks in no trumps, 10 tricks in hearts or spades, or 11 tricks in diamonds or clubs).

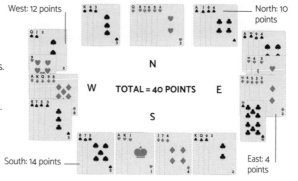

West: 12 points

North: 10 points

N

W   TOTAL = 40 POINTS   E

S

South: 14 points

East: 4 points

EXERCISE 3 | PLAY

Once bidding is over, play begins. The player who placed the winning bid becomes the declarer, and their partner is the dummy. The goal of the declaring pair is to match or make more than the number of tricks bid, and the goal of the opposing pair (the defenders) is to prevent them from doing so.

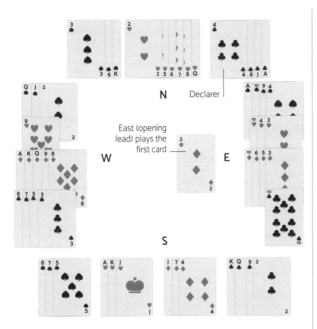

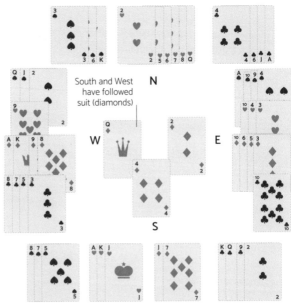

① The person to the left of the declarer plays the first card (the opening lead). This can be any card they like. The next player, the dummy, then places their cards faceup on the table and is no longer involved in the play. The dummy's partner, the declarer, will play both hands.

② Play continues clockwise around the table until four cards have been played. If they can, players must follow suit–play a card from the suit that has been led (in this case, diamonds). If all four players follow suit, the highest card played will win the trick.

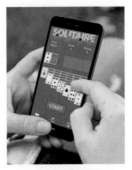
EXERCISE 4 | SCORING

Once 13 tricks have been played, both pairs count how many tricks they have won. The declaring side win points if they make their contract by achieving their target number of tricks, or more–but if they make fewer than predicted, the defenders score points instead (50 points for each trick by which the declarers are short of their target). If you are playing a friendly game, you will be playing rubber bridge, a "rubber" being the best of three games. When a pair has won a game by scoring 100 points or more, they become "vulnerable," and rewards and penalties increase. Part scores bid and made are carried forward, until one side passes 100.

Research has shown that regularly playing bridge improves reasoning skills and long- and short-term memory

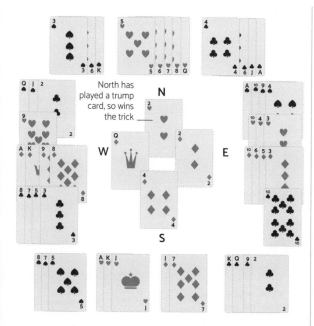

North has played a trump card, so wins the trick

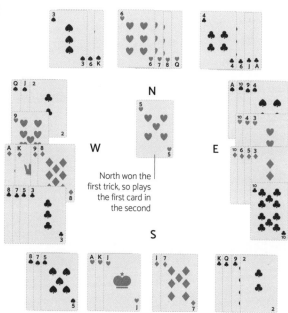

North won the first trick, so plays the first card in the second

③ If a player cannot follow suit, they may play—or "discard"—any card from another suit. Alternatively, if there is a trump suit (hearts, in this case), they can play a trump card. The highest trump card wins the trick—it trumps all other cards. This is known as "ruffing."

④ The player who won the trick opens the next trick, and can play any card in any suit. Play continues in this way until all 13 tricks have been played. Once scores have been calculated, the person to the left of the last dealer deals the next hand, and bidding begins again.

SCORING TABLE

No points are awarded for the first six tricks

A no-trump contract is the most valuable

Bidding and winning 13 tricks is called a "grand slam," and earns you bonus points (12 tricks is a "small slam")

Contracts above and to the right of this line are worth 100 points or more and result in "game" (extra tricks won do not count toward game)

If the declaring side win 11 tricks with hearts as trumps, they will score 150 points, plus any rewards

If you bid a contract that will earn you less than 100 points, this is called a "part score"

Tricks taken	1–6	7	8	9	10	11	12	13
No-trump **NT**		40	70	100	130	160	190	220
Spades ♠		30	60	90	120	150	180	210
Hearts ♥		30	60	90	120	150	180	210
Diamonds ♦		20	40	60	80	100	120	140
Clubs ♣		20	40	60	80	100	120	140

TRY POTTERY

Clay can be modeled into beautiful objects. Making pottery is a tactile, creative process, but it involves a lot of trial and error. Don't get discouraged–you can always squash your clay and start again!

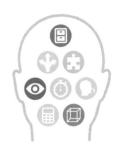

EXERCISE 1 | PINCH POT

Many pots are "thrown" using a wheel, but there are ways to construct a pot without committing to an expensive purchase. You don't even need true clay for your first experiments–air-dry or oven-dry modeling clays can be bought from any hobby shop.

PINCH POT

THINKING SKILLS

Boosts imagination and creativity

•

Improves concentration

•

Reduces stress

•

Improves fine motor skills in hands and fingers

---

(1) Roll a lump of clay in your hands until it is smooth and pliable.

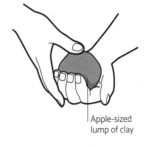

Apple-sized lump of clay

(2) Press a thumb into the center, leaving enough to clay form a base.

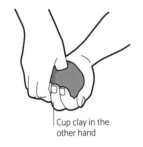

Cup clay in the other hand

(3) Squeeze the clay out between finger and thumb to form the walls.

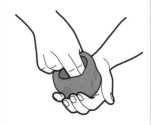

(4) Don't make the walls too thin, or they might collapse.

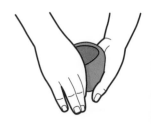

---

(5) Tamp the pot onto a flat surface to make a level base.

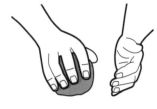

(6) You can smooth the outside of the walls if you want to.

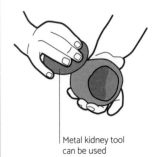

Metal kidney tool can be used

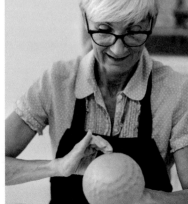

YOUR OWN STYLE

You can make a virtue of the uneven style of a pinched pot by arranging the pinch marks as a regular, decorative feature.

EXERCISE 2 | COILED POT

Another easy technique involves making a long rope of clay that is gradually piled around and up on itself to form the walls of the pot. Make a slab for the base. The first coil should be put on top of the slab rather than around its edge. The slab can be trimmed at the end. As the pot is coiled, you can smooth it inside and out.

COILED POT

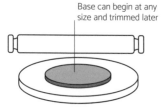

① Roll your clay into a slab for the base.

Base can begin at any size and trimmed later

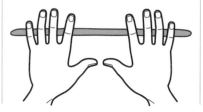

② Roll the clay into a rope around 1/4 in (5 mm) in diameter.

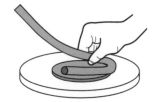

③ Place one end of the rope on the base and coil it.

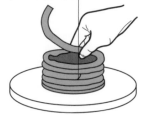

④ Lay a second coil on top, pushing down with your fingers to join it to the first.

Oblique join between coils

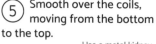

⑤ Smooth over the coils, moving from the bottom to the top.

Use a metal kidney tool if you have one

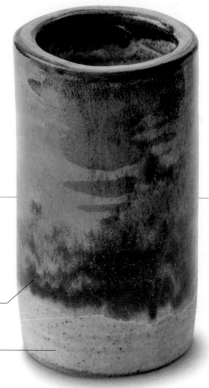

TAKE IT FURTHER

Your next steps might include decorating, glazing, and firing your pottery. But you can work with air-dry clay or polymer clay, neither of which needs firing, or metal clay, which can be fired with a blowtorch at home.

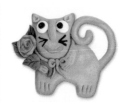

POLYMER CLAY MODEL

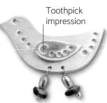

Toothpick impression

METAL CLAY BROOCH

Decorative pattern achieved with a mixture of glazes

Glossy, waterproof finish produced by melting glaze in kiln

SMOOTHED, GLAZED, AND FIRED COILED VASE

TRY SOME KNOTS

Knotting is a relatively simple skill with many practical applications, although knots are also good exercise for your brain and keep your fingers nimble.

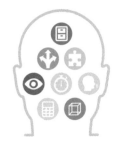

THINKING SKILLS

Improves 3-D visualization

Helps creativity and develops problem-solving skills

Improves eye-hand coordination

EXERCISE 1 | TURQUOISE TURTLE

Binding knots are commonly used to secure loose objects together or to wrap up both ends of the same rope. The turquoise turtle is an example of a binding knot and it is excellent for tying shoelaces, since it very rarely comes undone but is easy to release.

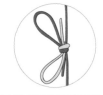

TURQUOISE TURTLE

---

(1) Loop one end around an object. Then make two turns around the standing (stationary) end.

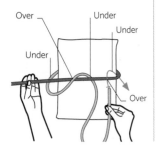

Over · Under · Under · Under · Over

(2) Hold the standing end firmly and pull the other end of the rope.

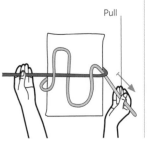

Pull

(3) Form two loops (called bights) by folding the two ends back on themselves.

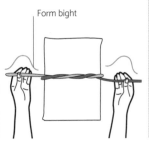

Form bight

(4) Bring the two bights together, crossing the right one over the left.

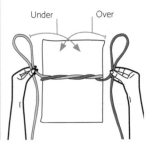

Under · Over

---

(5) Wrap the loop at the back around and over the front loop.

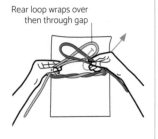

Rear loop wraps over then through gap

(6) The loop from the left and the loose end from the right now both go through the gap.

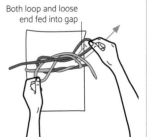

Both loop and loose end fed into gap

(7) The knot may look a bit messy now, but see what happens when you pull on both loops.

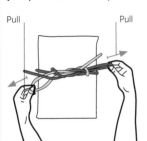

Pull · Pull

(8) Take a firm hold of the loops and pull them to tighten the knot.

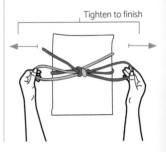

Tighten to finish

EXERCISE 2 | ROUND TURN AND TWO HALF HITCHES

This knot is commonly used for mooring a boat and can be used to attach a rope to a ring, pole, or other fixed support. It forms a reasonably strong bind, but can be untied even when there is a heavy load on the rope.

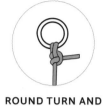

ROUND TURN AND TWO HALF HITCHES

The active end of a rope or line that moves to tie a knot is called the working end: the other is called the standing end

① To secure a rope to a ring, start by threading the working end behind and through the ring.

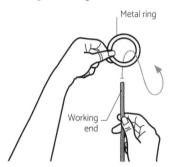

Metal ring

Working end

② To make the round turn, take the end of the rope behind the ring and thread it through again.

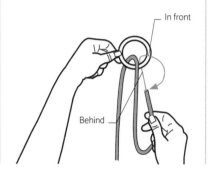

In front

Behind

③ To make the first half hitch, the working end travels first under and then over the standing end. Pull the working end to tighten the knot.

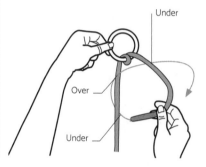

Under

Over

Under

④ Repeat the process in part 3 to make another half hitch, making sure that the half hitches are in the same direction.

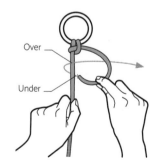

Over

Under

⑤ Hold on to the standing end to keep the line taut and then pull the working end to tighten the knot.

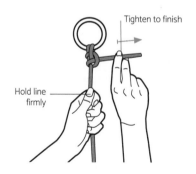

Tighten to finish

Hold line firmly

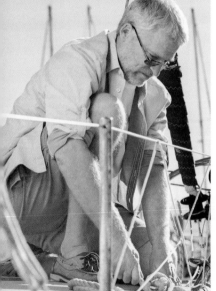

NECESSARY SKILL
Many different knots were developed for sailing, and hitch knots remain popular with sailors because they are quick to tie and also easy to undo.

EXERCISE 4 |
TIE A MONKEY'S FIST

This knot creates a stopper at the end of a rope to prevent the rope from slipping through an opening. It adds weight to a rope that needs to be thrown, but can also be ornamental, for example being used as a key fob.

MONKEY'S FIST

① Estimate the amount of rope you will need and then start by wrapping the rope around your hand.

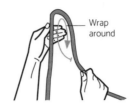

Wrap around

② Wrap the working end around your hand another two times.

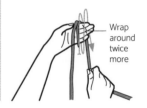

Wrap around twice more

③ Grip the loops with your thumb.

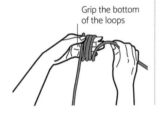

Grip the bottom of the loops

④ Turn your hand and wrap the rope around the loops.

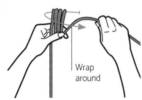

Wrap around

⑤ Working inward, wrap the rope around the loops two more times.

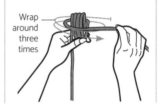

Wrap around three times

⑥ Pass the working end through the bottom and top of the first loops.

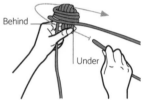

Behind

Under

⑦ Repeat Step 6 three more times.

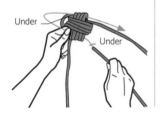

Under

Under

⑧ If you need to add weight to the knot, this can be inserted now.

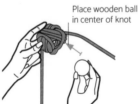

Place wooden ball in center of knot

⑨ Rotate the knot by 90° as you pull the rope through once more.

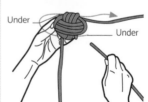

Under

Under

⑩ Pass the rope through the loops now facing the front

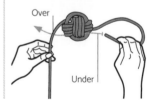

Over

Under

⑪ Hold the knot and pull on the working end to tighten the knot.

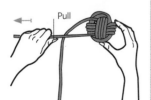

Pull

Pull

⑫ Work out the slack on the loops.

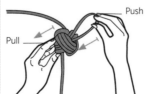

Push

Pull

⑬ Work the knot into an even shape while working out the slack.

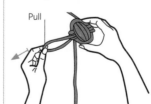

Pull

⑭ To finish, pull the ends to ensure the knot is tight.

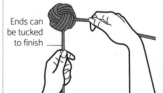

Ends can be tucked to finish

TAKE IT FURTHER

Once you've familiarized yourself with the basic knotting techniques, you can experiment with many types of knots and their practical applications. You can also explore knot-work further by looking at crafts, such as tatting and macramé (see below) that have developed to use rope, cord, or thread to create practical or decorative objects.

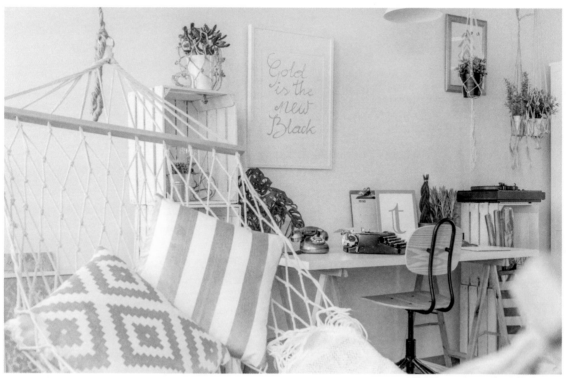

MACRAMÉ HAMMOCK

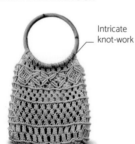

Intricate knot-work

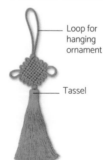

Loop for hanging ornament

Tassel

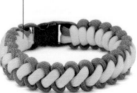

A bracelet is an easy way to carry around spare paracord

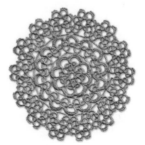

MACRAMÉ

Macramé is the art of tying knots to form loose textiles and is often used to create practical items, such as bags and plant hangers.

CHINESE DECORATIVE KNOTS

Knots as decoration have been around for thousands of years in China. The knots are usually symmetrical.

WEAVING WITH PARACORD

Tough and colorful cord, such as the cords used in parachutes, can be woven together to create bracelets.

TATTING

This old decorative skill uses simple knots, such as half-hitches, to create intricate patterns. It is often used to make lace collars and doilies.

TRY NEEDLECRAFTS

Needlecrafts such as knitting, sewing, and crochet are a relaxing way to counteract a busy day. At the same time, they stimulate the brain through eye–hand coordination, pattern following, concentration, and thinking ahead.

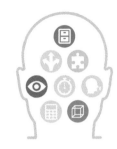

THINKING SKILLS

Relaxes the mind
·
Absorbing and creative
·
Enhances fine motor skills
·
Works memory

CHALLENGE 1 | EMBROIDER WITH CROSS-STITCH

Cross-stitch is one of the easiest embroidery techniques to learn. Kits provide you with everything you need to complete an item, or you can have fun shopping for notions and planning your own design.

① Bring the needle up through the fabric from behind.

② Insert the needle one space up and across from the first hole.

③ Bring the needle back up through the space under the second hole.

④ Take it across the first stitch to form a symmetrical cross.

Finished cross

Even-weave fabrics have regular spaces

First half of stitch

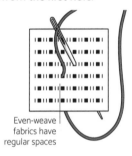
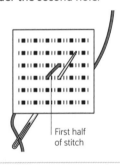
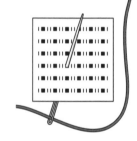
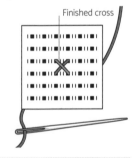

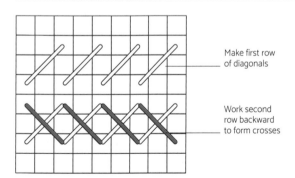

Make first row of diagonals

Work second row backward to form crosses

FILLING SPACE

Sometimes designs have a large area of the same color to fill. The quickest way to do this is to make a series of diagonal stitches along a row and then come back across them in the opposite direction.

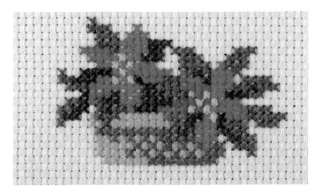

CREATE A PICTURE

Cross-stitch designs are created using a block of color for each stitch. Even though the designs look pixelated, this worked piece is clearly recognizable as a basket of poinsettias.

CHALLENGE 2 | CROCHET A BLANKET SQUARE

At its most basic, crochet involves forming interlocking loops with a hooked needle and yarn. Learn how to cast a chain and then practice making some simple stitches before you attempt an easy blanket, or "granny," square. This pattern involves three stitches: chain, slip, and double.

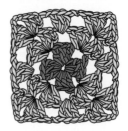

FINISHED SQUARE

(1) Start with a slipknot. Wrap the yarn around the hook to form a loop and pull the yarn through.

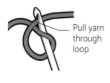

Pull yarn through loop

Slide knot up to tighten

(2) Wrap the yarn around the hook and draw it through to make the first chain. Make four more.

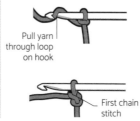

Pull yarn through loop on hook

First chain stitch

(3) Form the chains into a ring by making a slip stitch into the first chain after the slipknot.

Hook yarn and pull straight through chain and stitch on hook

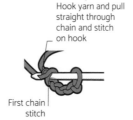

First chain stitch

(4) Make three chain to start the next row (this also acts as the first of three doubles–see panel for how to make these).

Three chain coming up from ring

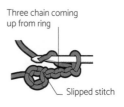

Slipped stitch

(5) For a blanket square, work two doubles (see panel) into the ring.

Make three chain after second double

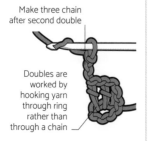

Doubles are worked by hooking yarn through ring rather than through a chain

(6) Repeat sequence of three chain and three doubles until you have four groups of doubles.

Slip stitch into third chain of first group to close round

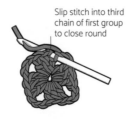

(7) Start the second row with three chain and make two double groups into the first corner.

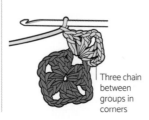

Three chain between groups in corners

(8) Repeat into the other three corners and slip stitch to finish. Add more rows as required.

Make one chain before starting next group

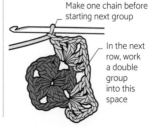

In the next row, work a double group into this space

HOW TO MAKE A DOUBLE

(1) To make a double stitch, wrap the yarn around the hook and push it into the fourth chain.

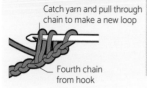

Catch yarn and pull through chain to make a new loop

Fourth chain from hook

(2) Wrap the yarn around the hook and pull it through the first two loops on the hook.

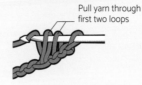

Pull yarn through first two loops

(3) Catch the yarn again and pull it through the two remaining loops to leave one loop on hook.

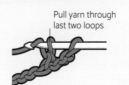

Pull yarn through last two loops

(4) A finished double should look like this. Repeat steps 1, 2, and 3 to make a new double.

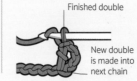

Finished double

New double is made into next chain

CHALLENGE 3 | KNIT A SCARF

Knitting is undergoing one of its periodical revivals. It's not hard to see why—it keeps your fingers busy, takes your mind off other things, and you end up with a unique handmade item at the end. Once you learn how to manipulate the needles and yarn, cast on and off, and master a few basic techniques and stitches, you can make anything. Why not start with a simple, easy-knit scarf?

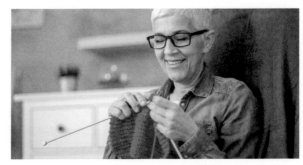

CREATE A COZY SCARF

① CAST ON

To start knitting, you need to put stitches onto a needle, a process called casting on. There are at least six ways to cast on, but this method shows you how to do it by knitting into the first stitch on the needle. Start by making a slipknot and tighten it onto a needle. Cast on enough stitches to give you a decent-width scarf.

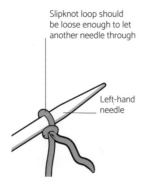

Slipknot loop should be loose enough to let another needle through

Left-hand needle

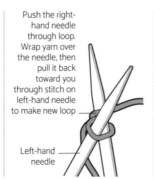

Push the right-hand needle through loop. Wrap yarn over the needle, then pull it back toward you through stitch on left-hand needle to make new loop

Left-hand needle

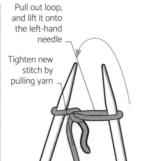

Pull out loop, and lift it onto the left-hand needle

Tighten new stitch by pulling yarn

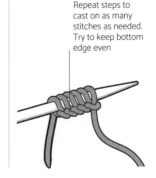

Repeat steps to cast on as many stitches as needed. Try to keep bottom edge even

② KNIT STITCH

The most basic stitch is the knit or plain stitch. Put the empty needle through the bottom of the first stitch on the needle. Wrap the yarn around the needle and pull it through, taking the stitch onto the empty needle. Repeat until all the stitches are transferred. Swap the needles over and start the next row.

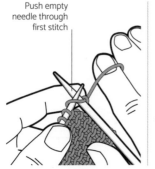

Push empty needle through first stitch

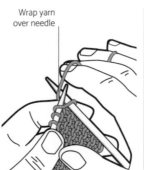

Wrap yarn over needle

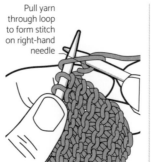

Pull yarn through loop to form stitch on right-hand needle

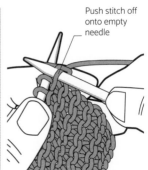

Push stitch off onto empty needle

③ ADD IN COLOR

Continue knitting rows of plain stitch until you reach the required length for your scarf. If you prefer a striped scarf you can add a new color at the start of a row by knitting it into the first stitch. Hold on tightly to the new color until you have made a few stitches, then cut off a length of the first color. The tails of the two yarns can be darned in later.

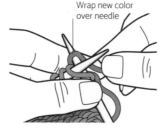

Wrap new color over needle

START A NEW COLOR

Start with short, medium-sized needles and an Aran or DK weight yarn. Very thick, fine, or long needles are hard to hold when you are learning. Experiment with holding needles and yarn together until they feel easy

④ CAST OFF

To finish your work, the stitches have to be cast off so they don't unravel. Knit the first two stitches, then lift the first stitch over the second. Knit another stitch, then lift the previous stitch over it. Repeat until one stitch is left on the right needle, then cut the yarn, thread it through the loop, and pull tight.

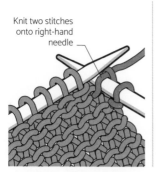

Knit two stitches onto right-hand needle

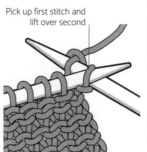

Pick up first stitch and lift over second

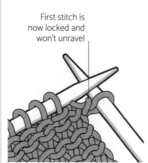

First stitch is now locked and won't unravel

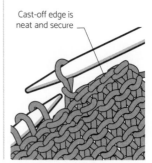

Cast-off edge is neat and secure

TAKE IT FURTHER

CROCHET

There are many other patterns for blanket squares. Learn new stitches and patterns from online tutorials. Then try making a garment such as a hat or a scarf.

KNITTING

Learn how to do purl and slip stitches, and how to increase and decrease, which are key to shaping. Then try some easy patterns, such as stockinette stitch, rib, and seed stitch. You could even try arm knitting (without needles).

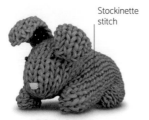

Stockinette stitch

TOY RABBIT

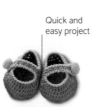

Quick and easy project

CROCHETED BABY BOOTIES

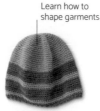

Learn how to shape garments

CROCHETED BEANIE HAT

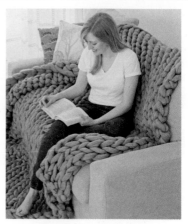

ARM KNITTING CREATES CHUNKY-KNIT TEXTILES

TRY ORIGAMI AND PAPER CRAFT

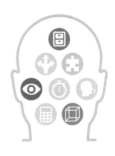

Origami is the ancient Japanese art of paper folding. By simply turning and folding the paper you can create objects for any occasion. Special origami paper is thin, square, and has a different color or pattern on each side, but you can practice with any sheet of paper you have on hand.

CHALLENGE 1 | **FOLD A FOX**

Try your hand at this fantastic fox to give you a taste for origami. He will look even better if you use a paper that is red or orange on one side and white on the other. No gluing or cutting is allowed–the origami discipline is confined to folding.

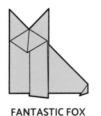

FANTASTIC FOX

① Fold paper along red dashed line

② Fold in half again and open out

③ Fold both outer points up to the top point so that edges meet in the middle

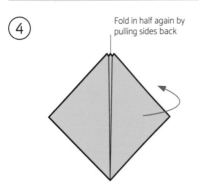

④ Fold in half again by pulling sides back

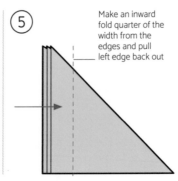

⑤ Make an inward fold quarter of the width from the edges and pull left edge back out

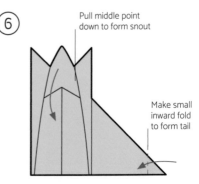

⑥ Pull middle point down to form snout

Make small inward fold to form tail

CHALLENGE 2 | SIMPLE SWAN

This graceful swan is easy to fold. Try making it with crisp paper napkins and have a flock of swans swimming down your dining table for a special occasion.

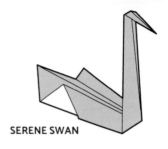
SERENE SWAN

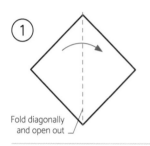
① Fold diagonally and open out

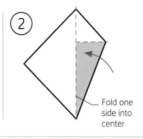
② Fold one side into center

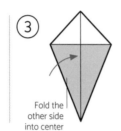
③ Fold the other side into center

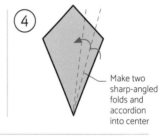
④ Make two sharp-angled folds and accordion into center

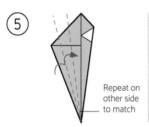
⑤ Repeat on other side to match

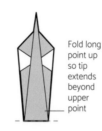
⑥ Fold long point up so tip extends beyond upper point

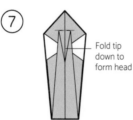
⑦ Fold tip down to form head

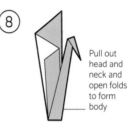
⑧ Pull out head and neck and open folds to form body

CHALLENGE 3 | PERFECT A PIG

This little pig is more of a challenge, but if you follow the diagram carefully you will soon start to anticipate where the folds need to be made and where to push them in to create the nose and tail.

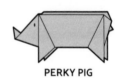
PERKY PIG

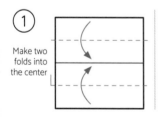
① Make two folds into the center

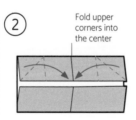
② Fold upper corners into the center

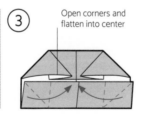
③ Open corners and flatten into center

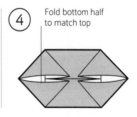
④ Fold bottom half to match top

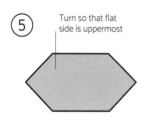
⑤ Turn so that flat side is uppermost

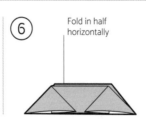
⑥ Fold in half horizontally

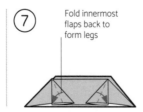
⑦ Fold innermost flaps back to form legs

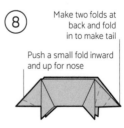
⑧ Make two folds at back and fold in to make tail

Push a small fold inward and up for nose

CHALLENGE 4 | FUNKY FROG

Take your newly acquired origami skills up a notch with this funky green frog. When you've finished, you can make him jump by pressing down gently on the bottom folds. Why not make a few and have a competition to see whose frog can jump farthest?

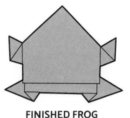

FINISHED FROG

① Fold in half horizontally and open out

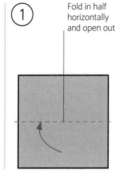

② Fold in half vertically

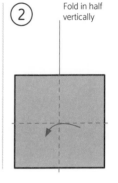

⑧ Push in sides along fold lines and flatten into point

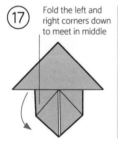

⑨ Turn up bottom of paper to meet base of triangle

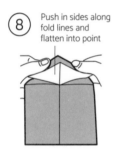

⑩ Fold left hand side of paper in half under triangle

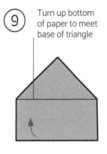

⑪ Repeat on right hand side

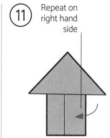

⑫ Fold up bottom half of rectangle to meet base of triangle

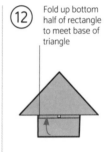

⑰ Fold the left and right corners down to meet in middle

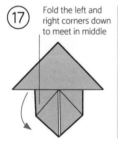

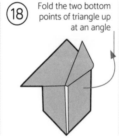

⑱ Fold the two bottom points of triangle up at an angle

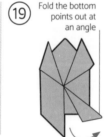

⑲ Fold the bottom points out at an angle

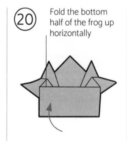

⑳ Fold the bottom half of the frog up horizontally

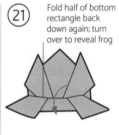

㉑ Fold half of bottom rectangle back down again; turn over to reveal frog

CHALLENGE 5 | BOX SMART

Making boxes is not the same as origami, but it presents an interesting spatial and mathematical challenge. Templates are available on the Internet, but designing your own and figuring out how to cut and fold the card stock will give your brain a workout. Use colored or printed card stock for a more luxurious look.

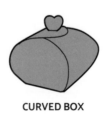

CURVED BOX

① Make a slit at both ends wide enough for tabs

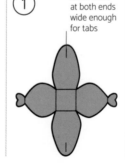

② Bring tabbed ends together, then pass slitted ends over them to fasten

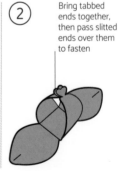

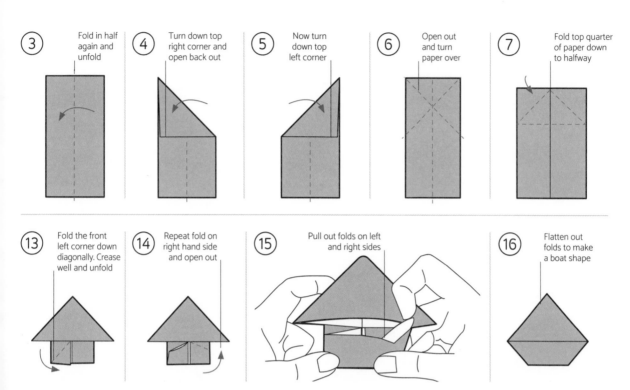

③ Fold in half again and unfold

④ Turn down top right corner and open back out

⑤ Now turn down top left corner

⑥ Open out and turn paper over

⑦ Fold top quarter of paper down to halfway

⑬ Fold the front left corner down diagonally. Crease well and unfold

⑭ Repeat fold on right hand side and open out

⑮ Pull out folds on left and right sides

⑯ Flatten out folds to make a boat shape

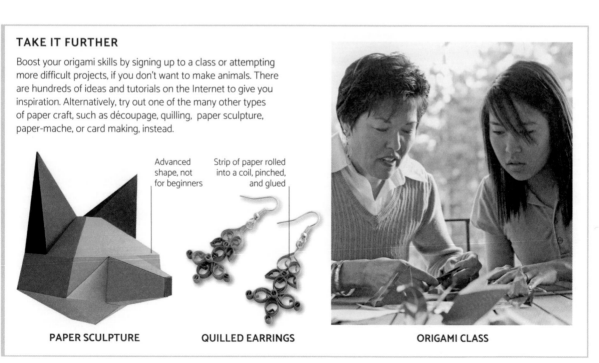

TAKE IT FURTHER

Boost your origami skills by signing up to a class or attempting more difficult projects, if you don't want to make animals. There are hundreds of ideas and tutorials on the Internet to give you inspiration. Alternatively, try out one of the many other types of paper craft, such as découpage, quilling, paper sculpture, paper-mache, or card making, instead.

Advanced shape, not for beginners

Strip of paper rolled into a coil, pinched, and glued

PAPER SCULPTURE

QUILLED EARRINGS

ORIGAMI CLASS

TRY GARDENING

Gardening is a deeply satisfying hobby. Watching something you have planted grow inspires a great sense of achievement, even if you only have a balcony or a small outdoor space.

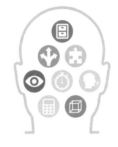

CHALLENGE 1 | **PICTURE THIS**

Succulents are great plants for the beginner. They come in a wide range of shapes, colors, and habits, and they require relatively little maintenance. Garden centers keep succulents all year round. Choose flat rather than tall varieties to stop them from falling out.

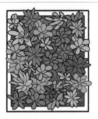

HANGING GARDEN

THINKING SKILLS

Reduces stress

•

Boosts immunity

•

Increases self-esteem, motivation, and satisfaction

•

Enhances mood and connection with nature

① Choose a deep picture frame or shallow box. Paint or varnish, then fix a hook to the back for hanging.

Needs weather-resistant paint or varnish

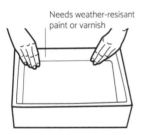

② Attach a layer of strong plastic (an old garbage bag is ideal) to the inside using a glue gun or staples and trim to fit.

Attach plastic to sides

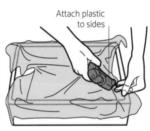

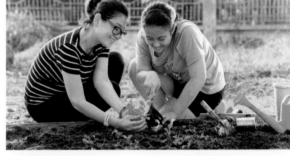

EAT YOUR GARDEN

If you have space, set up a vegetable patch. Tomatoes, carrots, and lettuce can also be grown in pots and taste better than store-bought.

③ Fill the frame with damp sphagnum moss from a garden center, making sure it is packed in with an even thickness.

Don't leave gaps, especially at corners

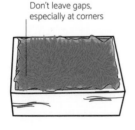

④ Staple or nail some chicken wire over the sphagnum and cut off the excess. Tuck in any sharp wire edges.

Stretch wire taught

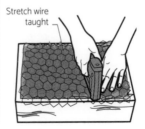

⑤ Carefully trim the roots of your plants, avoiding any taproots. Make holes in the moss and push the plants in.

Gaps can be filled with moss

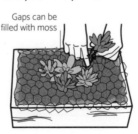

⑥ Leave your frame horizontal for 2 weeks to establish the plants, then hang or prop it against a wall.

When moss feels dry, take down and water lightly

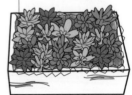

CHALLENGE 2 | MAKE A SPLASH

Water attracts wildlife to a garden. It doesn't have to be a large pond or stream—a large pot or trough will entice insects to set up home and provide somewhere for birds to bathe and drink.

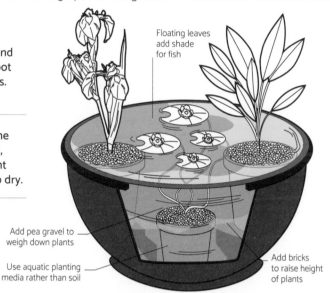

① Choose a large and sturdy ceramic pot without drainage holes. Move into place.

② If the inside of the pot is not glazed, paint with pond sealant and leave overnight to dry.

③ Fill the pot with water and check for leaks and seepage. Reseal if necessary.

Floating leaves add shade for fish

Add pea gravel to weigh down plants

Use aquatic planting media rather than soil

Add bricks to raise height of plants

④ Select a mixture of aquatic and bog plants that help oxygenate the water.

⑤ If you plan to add fish, leave the pot to stand for at least a week to dechlorinate the water.

⑥ Remove dead plant material regularly. Empty the pot and remove plants and fish in winter to prevent freezing.

CHALLENGE 3 | TAKE ON A PROJECT

Is there an area of your yard that you would like to improve? Why not make some plans now? Make "before" and "after" sketches and anticipate how it will look in 2 or 5 years' time. Before reaching for the shovel, make a mood board of ideas, draw up a plan, source materials, and cost it. Then get digging!

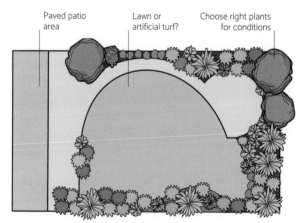

Paved patio area

Lawn or artificial turf?

Choose right plants for conditions

"AFTER" SKETCH OF YOUR IDEAL YARD

TAKE IT FURTHER

Gardening doesn't have to be a solo activity. Taking cuttings of plants in your garden and swapping them with neighbors is a cheap way to get more plants and it gets you involved in the community. You could also enter local competitions, such as flower and produce shows. Try growing a monster vegetable if you want a real challenge.

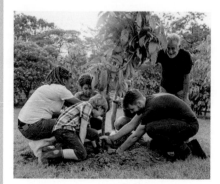

JOIN A COMMUNITY GARDEN PROJECT

TRY IDENTIFYING WILDFLOWERS

Wildflowers may grow on almost any patch of natural land. Learning to identify them will enhance your walks as well as improve your memory and observational skills.

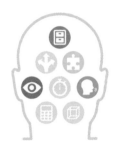

EXERCISE 1 | NAME THAT FLOWER

Identifying a wildflower draws upon your skills of observation. The best time to go flower spotting is in the spring and summer, when the flowers are out. At other times of the year, you have to rely on leaf shape, habit, seed heads, or buds.

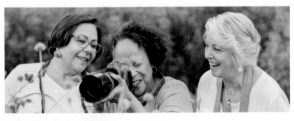

CAPTURE THE MOMENT
Photographing flowers is not just a good way to keep a record of species you've seen, it also lets you practise your photography skills.

(1) **WHAT TO SEE?** Different species thrive in different habitats, and it is useful to have an idea of what flowers you may see when you go for a walk. Take a field guide when you go out, or first familiarize yourself with flowers you are likely to see.

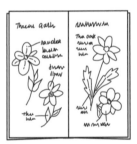

EXERCISE 2 | PRESS FLOWERS

Pressed flowers can be used to decorate items such as cards and candles. Keep freshly picked flowers in a sealable plastic bag until you get home, and then put them into water with a little sugar or flower food. Do not pick flowers in nature preserves or public parks.

(1) Space your flowers over one half-page of blotting paper. Make sure that they do not touch each other.

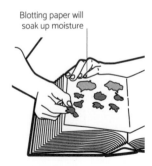

Blotting paper will soak up moisture

(2) Fold the paper over the flowers. Hold in place as you close the book. Add more flowers between other pages.

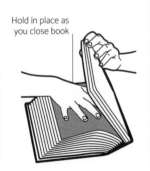

Hold in place as you close book

(3) Put some heavy books on top of the first one and leave to dry in a warm, dry place for about 4 weeks.

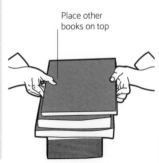

Place other books on top

② TAKE A CLOSER LOOK

All the parts of the flower have a role in fertilization. Take a careful look at a flower to count the number of male reproductive parts (stamens) and petals arranged around the female parts, as that may aid in identifying the species.

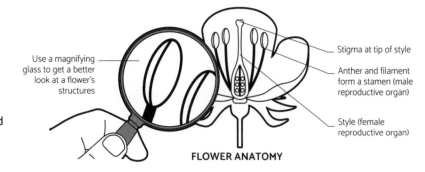

Use a magnifying glass to get a better look at a flower's structures

Stigma at tip of style

Anther and filament form a stamen (male reproductive organ)

Style (female reproductive organ)

FLOWER ANATOMY

③ IDENTIFYING FEATURES

The shape of a flower, the number of petals, as well as its color, make some species easy to identify. Plants may have solitary flowers or flowers arranged in clusters. If a plant has no flowers, seeds and fruit provide vital clues to its identity.

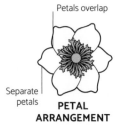
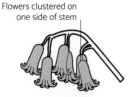
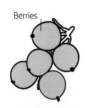

Petals overlap

Separate petals

PETAL ARRANGEMENT

Flowers clustered on one side of stem

FLOWER ARRANGEMENT

Berries

FRUITS AND SEEDS

④ KEEP A RECORD

Make notes of the flowers you find and record any relevant details that may help to identify the species. You can also sketch or take photos of the flowers you observe so that you can identify them later. Detailed records let you create a database of what species you saw and when.

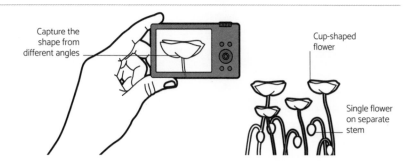

Capture the shape from different angles

Cup-shaped flower

Single flower on separate stem

④

To stick a flower onto a card, hold it with tweezers and apply a dab of glue to the back of it with a toothpick.

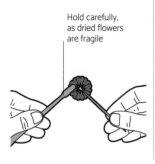

Hold carefully, as dried flowers are fragile

⑤

Use tweezers to position the flower on the card. Press gently with the tweezers to firm the flower down.

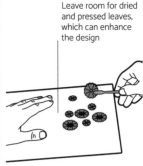

Leave room for dried and pressed leaves, which can enhance the design

⑥

Leave the finished picture to dry. If you want, seal the flowers in place with sticky or iron-on transparent film.

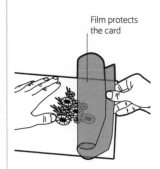

Film protects the card

TAKE IT FURTHER

Wildflowers are part of important ecosystems. The insects that are drawn to specific species of flower may help to identify the plant, but are also worth a closer look themselves.

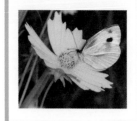

GET CLOSER TO TREES

Trees can be found in most habitats, and you can improve your knowledge and observation skills by discovering how to identify the species in your neighborhood.

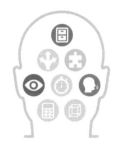

EXERCISE | TAKE A GOOD LOOK

Pick a tree you don't know. Now start asking yourself some questions. Throughout the year, observe the tree's bark, buds, leaves, flowers, and fruit (if it has them), and see if you can link them all together to build a complete picture of the species. Take notes and photographs if you're out in the field.

(1) **TREE MEASURING**
The height and spread of a tree are useful identifying traits. Have a friend stand beneath the tree and use a pencil to estimate height and width by comparing these measurements to your friend's height.

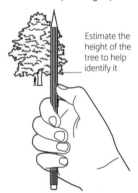

Estimate the height of the tree to help identify it

(2) **BARK RUBBING**
If you can't draw the bark of a tree, make a rubbing of it so that you can have an accurate record of the texture.

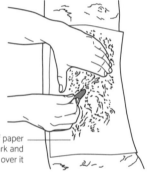

Place a piece of paper against the bark and rub crayon over it

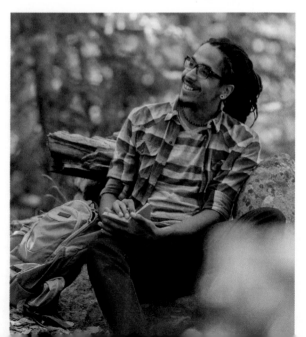

(3) **KEEP A RECORD**
Build up a record, and do this for several, or many, different species, building your knowledge into a datafile on cards, a computer database, or simply a nature notebook.

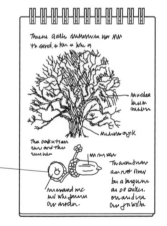

Sketch and make notes of the details you observe

MOOD AND MEMORY
Spending time in nature may help improve your mood, but you can also use the time to sharpen your memory by learning to identify species.

④ LEAF SHAPES
The size and shape of a plant's leaves enable the plant to thrive in its natural habitat and climate.

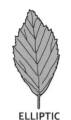 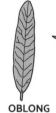 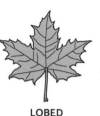 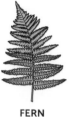 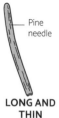 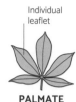

ELLIPTIC   OBLONG   LOBED   FERN

Pine needle

LONG AND THIN

Individual leaflet

PALMATE (HAND-SHAPED)

⑤ LEAF MARGINS
The edges of leaves can tell you about the plant and its natural environment. Smooth margins help a plant to lose less moisture than toothed edges.

No serration or indentation   Rounded indentations   Lots of fine serrations   Forward-pointing teeth   Undulating edges   Protection against pests

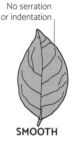 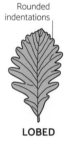 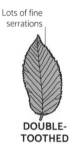 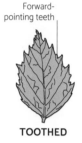 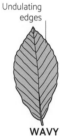 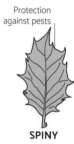

SMOOTH   LOBED   DOUBLE-TOOTHED   TOOTHED   WAVY   SPINY

⑥ LEAF ARRANGEMENT
The leaves can be arranged in many different ways. Make a note of the arrangement, since it provides clues to a tree's identity.

Flattened sprays

Leaves on a central axis

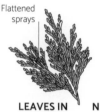 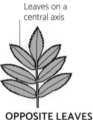 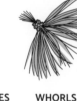 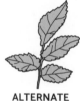

LEAVES IN CLUSTERS   NEEDLE LEAVES ON A SHOOT   OPPOSITE LEAVES   WHORLS   ALTERNATE LEAVES

⑦ DOES IT HAVE FRUITS OR SEEDS?
From midsummer, you can see trees forming fruits and seeds that, in cool latitudes, will drop to the ground in the fall.

Seeds are dispersed by wind

May be dispersed by animals

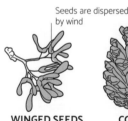 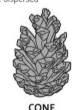

WINGED SEEDS   CONE   EDIBLE FRUIT

⑧ DOES IT HAVE FLOWERS?
Many trees have flowers that will help to identify the species. The shapes of the flowers can tell you how the flowers are pollinated.

Colored petals

Reproductive organs

Hanging male flowers

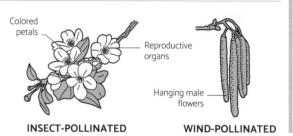

INSECT-POLLINATED   WIND-POLLINATED

TAKE IT FURTHER

Look at what is growing around, on, or in trees. Trees have their own little ecosystem of animals, plants, and fungi that depend on them for food and shelter. Make a special trip in the fall to see how the leaf colors change on some trees. Keep a journal and mark the changes. Enhance your yard by planting a tree. Think about its size, habit, and suitability for the plot. Then enjoy it changing and growing over the years. Try photographing trees in different seasons, light, and times of day.

TRY BIRDWATCHING

Birdwatching is one of the most accessible ways to view wild animals and it can be done almost anywhere. Learning to identify birds will sharpen your memory and your observational skills.

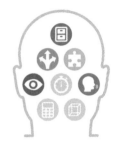

EXERCISE 1 | ATTRACT BIRDS

Birds will visit almost any green space, but if you plan to attract regular visitors to somewhere you can watch them, such as a backyard or balcony, consider their needs. Ideally you should provide food, the right nesting conditions, plants for cover, and water. If you do not have the space, a feeder can be stuck to a window.

1 FEEDERS
Choose a feeder for the type of birds you want to attract. Place feeders away from where predators can hide.

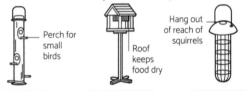

Perch for small birds — **TUBE FEEDER**

Roof keeps food dry — **TABLE FEEDER**

Hang out of reach of squirrels — **SUET FEEDER**

2 PLANTS
Flowers and fruits may provide food for some species, but also attract insects that many backyard birds feed on.

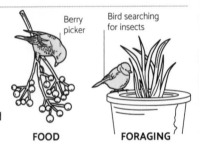

Berry picker

Bird searching for insects

FOOD

FORAGING

3 WATER
A source of water is not just a place for drinking. Birds will also use a birdbath as a place to groom themselves.

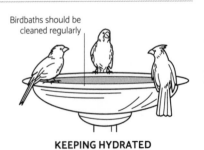

Birdbaths should be cleaned regularly

KEEPING HYDRATED

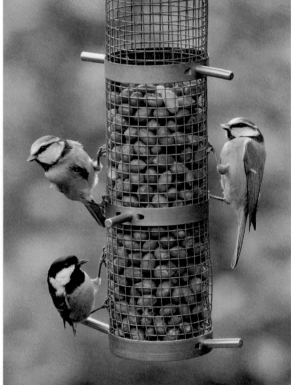

FEEDING TOGETHER
It is not unusual to see different species visiting the same feeder, although during mating season birds may become more territorial and chase away other birds.

EXERCISE 2 | PLUMAGE

A bird's feathers give a species distinctive colors and markings. The largest group of birds in the world is the passerines (perching birds), and while birds in passerine families may be similar in size and shape, they often have distinguishing markings that help identify them. Use the illustration to the right to familiarize yourself with the different plumage regions of a typical bird.

Crown
Supercilium
Nape
Lores
Throat
Malar region
Auriculars
Sides
Breast
Mantle
Rump
Uppertail corvets
Belly
Tail
Vent
Wing
Flanks

PLUMAGE REGIONS

① **FINE MARKINGS**
Study each bird here–paying attention to its distinguishing features–then turn to p.150 for Step 2.

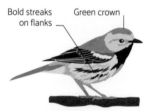

Bold streaks on flanks
Green crown

BLACK-THROATED GREEN WARBLER

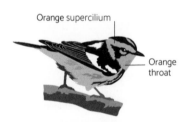

Orange supercilium
Orange throat

BLACKBURNIAN WARBLER

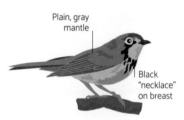

Plain, gray mantle
Black "necklace" on breast

CANADA WARBLER

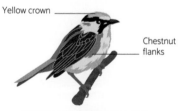

Yellow crown
Chestnut flanks

CHESTNUT-SIDED WARBLER

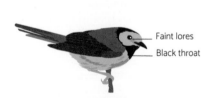

Faint lores
Black throat

HOODED WARBLER

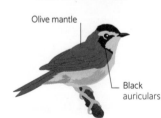

Olive mantle
Black auriculars

KENTUCKY WARBLER

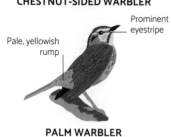

Prominent eyestripe
Pale, yellowish rump

PALM WARBLER

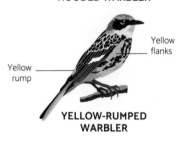

Yellow flanks
Yellow rump

YELLOW-RUMPED WARBLER

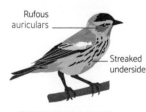

Rufous auriculars
Streaked underside

CAPE MAY WARBLER

② IDENTIFY THE BIRDS

These are the same birds that appear on p.149. Identify these birds by the highlighted colors and markings.

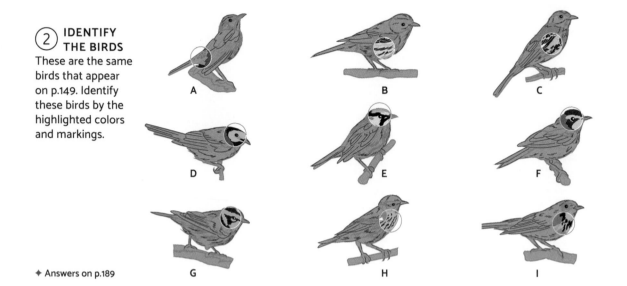

A   B   C

D   E   F

G   H   I

✦ Answers on p.189

EXERCISE 3 | KEEP A RECORD

You can use field guides to help you identify birds, but keeping a notebook will help you work your brain in many different ways. Pay careful attention to the different calls and songs of a bird, the way it flies, and any other behavior in order to train your eyes and ears to recognize a bird's distinguishing features.

① DRAW

Sketching birds will help you remember the details of those you spot. You can start with the overall shape of the bird, the size and shape of its bill, and the length of its tail. Then start to fill in the markings.

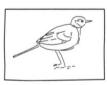

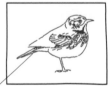

Add as many details as you can see

② SOUNDS

In some habitats, it may be hard to spot some birds, and getting to know their songs and calls will help you identify birds even when you cannot see them. Try to describe the various sounds you hear phonetically.

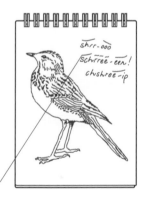

shrr-ooo
Schrree-een!
chshree-ip

Add lines to indicate rising or falling pitch and volume

③ FLIGHT PATTERNS

Identifying flying birds can be challenging, but make a note of the rhythm with which a bird flaps its wings, its wing shape, tail shape, and any patterns or color on the underwing.

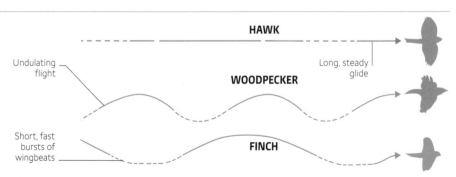

HAWK

Long, steady glide

Undulating flight

WOODPECKER

Short, fast bursts of wingbeats

FINCH

EXERCISE 4 | PLAN A TRIP

One of the joys of birdwatching is that you do not necessarily have to go far to see a variety of birds. Even in large cities, birds can be spotted in parks and squares. And the migration of birds means that there are seasonal variations in the species you are likely to see.

(1) PLAN
Whether you're going far or staying close to home, do some research to find out what birds you are likely to see when. Look at birding websites to find the ideal place to spot birds.

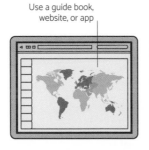
Use a guide book, website, or app

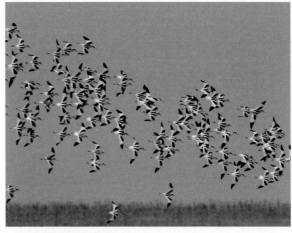

REWARDING HABITATS
A bird's habitat influences the likelihood of spotting it. Birds in forests or wooded areas may be solitary and harder to spot, but water birds live where it is harder for them to hide, so they often form flocks.

(2) WHAT TO PACK
You do not need a lot of equipment, but it is a good idea to carry a notebook with you always. A pair of binoculars may also come in handy.

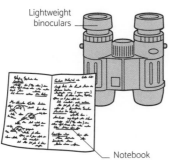
Lightweight binoculars

Notebook

(3) BLINDS
Wild birds are easily scared off by potential threats. A bird blind or a viewing platform gives birdwatchers a place to sit and wait for birds.

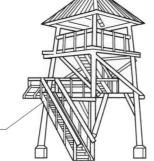
Viewing platform to spot wetland birds from a distance

TAKE IT FURTHER

If you become more serious about birding, you may want to consider investing in some equipment, such as a spotting scope or sound recording equipment. You can make birdwatching a more social experience by joining other birders on a chase or birding outing.

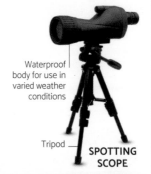
Waterproof body for use in varied weather conditions

Tripod

SPOTTING SCOPE

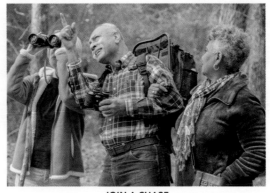
JOIN A CHASE

The world's top birders have seen more than 9,000 species

TRY STARGAZING

Stargazing tests your memory and hones your visual problem-solving skills. Learn to find some famous stars in the night sky and then use those stars to navigate to other interesting sights.

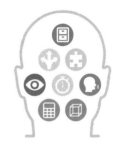

EXERCISE 1 | **HOPS FROM ORION**

The night sky is divided into 88 distinct areas, called constellations. Each constellation contains a figure made up of imaginary lines linking stars. Orion (the Hunter) is one of the best known constellations and is easily found by looking for the three bright stars that make up Orion's Belt. Orion is facing a Bull (Taurus).

① **TO THE DOG STAR**
Trace a line through the three stars in the belt, starting on the same side as Rigel. This line will soon reach Sirius (the Dog Star), the brightest star in the night sky.

② **TO A RED GIANT**
Extend the imaginary line in the opposite direction from step 1. The destination is the bright red star Aldebaran–the "eye" of Taurus.

③ **TO THE TWINS**
Follow an almost straight line from Rigel, through Betelgeuse, until you reach Castor in Gemini, the Twins. Nearby is Castor's slightly brighter twin, Pollux.

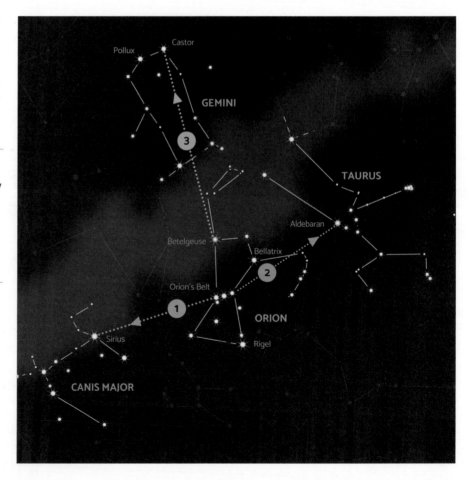

EXERCISE 2 | **NORTH NAVIGATION**

In the far north of the sky–a region of the celestial sphere visible only to stargazers in the northern hemisphere–are two particularly famous sights. Polaris (the North Star or Pole Star) was an important navigational aid for sailors, since true north lies directly below this star. The other famous figure in the northern sky is the seven-star pattern in Ursa Major (the Bear), known as the Big Dipper.

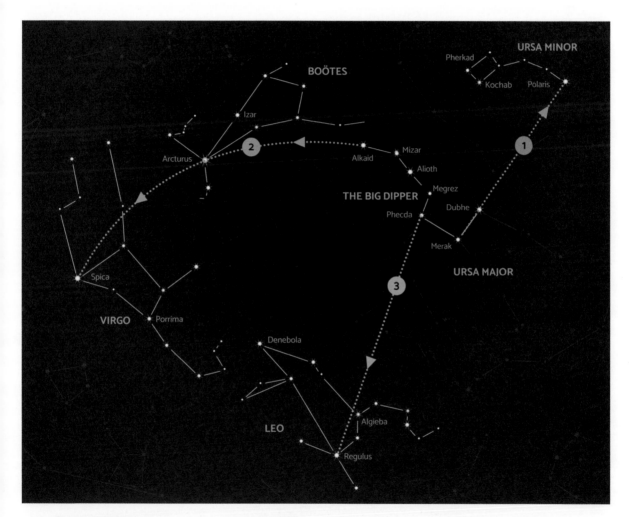

① **TO THE NORTH STAR**
Find the Big Dipper, which is shaped like a saucepan. Draw a line between the last two stars in the "bowl" (Merak and Dubhe) and extend the line to reach the North Star.

② **TO VIRGO**
The Big Dipper's handle is not straight and you can trace a curved path from the last three stars in the Big Dipper (Alioth, Mizar, and Alkaid), through Arcturus in Boötes, to reach Spica in Virgo.

③ **TO LEO**
To find the constellation Leo (the Lion), start at Megrez and draw a line to Phecda (also called Phad) at the base of the Big Dipper's "bowl." Continue this line out all the way to Regulus, a bright star in Leo.

EXERCISE 3 | SOUTHERN STAR HOPPING

The Southern Cross, or Crux, is the smallest of the 88 constellations. It is one of the most well-known constellations in the southern hemisphere, but is not visible to observers in the northern hemisphere. Crux sits near Rigil Kentaurus, the third brightest star in the night sky.

① THE SOUTHERN POINTERS

Find the Southern Cross. Start at the faintest of its four stars, Delta Crucis, and extend a line through Beta Crucis, opposite, until you reach the bright star Hadar and then the even brighter Rigil Kentaurus. Rigil Kentaurus and Hadar are known as the Southern Pointers because they can be used to locate the South Celestial Pole.

② TO THE SOUTH POLE

Draw a line between Hadar and Rigil Kentaurus, and then extend a bisecting line at a right angle to that line. Extend the axis of Crux. The South Celestial Pole is the point where these two lines cross.

③ THE SOUTHERN TRIANGLE

Extend a line from Al Birdhaun, through Rigil Kentaurus to the next fairly bright star, which is Atria. Atria is the brightest star in the constellation Triangulum Australe, the Southern Triangle.

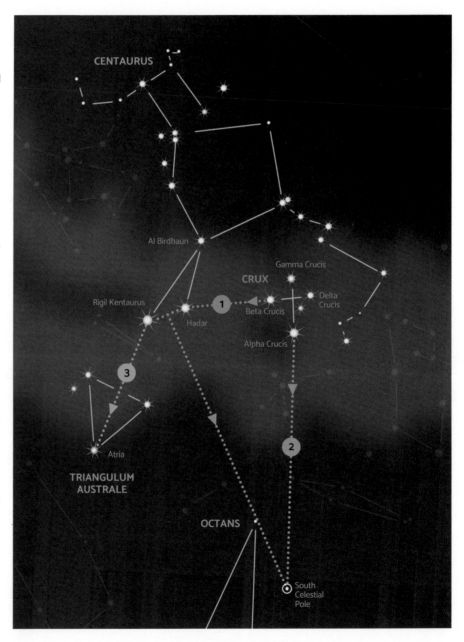

EXERCISE 4 | LUNAR LANDMARKS

On a clear night during (or near to) a full moon, mares (so named because they were once thought to be seas) and some craters on the near side of the moon are clearly visible.

(1) **LEARN**
Use the illustration on the right to memorize 12 surface features.

(2) **TEST**
Cover up the illustration and name the features (A–K) on the photo.

(3) **PRACTISE**
Do the same exercise looking at the moon on a clear night.

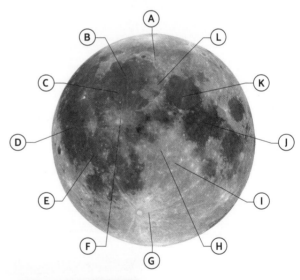

Plato
Mare Imbrium
Archimedes
Appennine
Mare Serenitatis
Copernicus
Kepler
Mare Tranquillitatis
Oceanus Procellarum
Ptolemaeus
Albategnius
Tycho

TAKE IT FURTHER

Even with modestly priced equipment it is possible to explore the night sky's magnificent sights. Setting up a telescope and taking photos of the night sky will mean having to learn some new skills, such as using coordinates to locate distant objects and compensating for the Earth's rotation.

Refractor telescope

Motorized mount keeps pace with Earth's spin

TELESCOPE

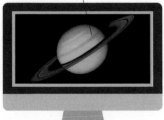

Composite digital image of Saturn

ASTROPHOTOGRAPHY
Taking photos of celestial objects, such as galaxies and planets, is made easier with image-processing software that helps to combine multiple exposures to create a single, clear photograph.

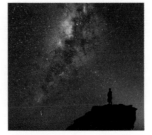

THE NAKED EYE
You don't need expensive equipment to explore the night sky. Away from the interference of artificial light, many celestial bodies and phenomena, such as the Milky Way, can be seen with the naked eye.

TRY TENNIS

Tennis is a great way to get some physical and mental exercise. The goal is to out-think and outlast your opponent by using placement, power, and spin to stop them from returning the ball.

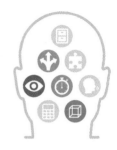

EXERCISE 1 | GROUNDSTROKES

The basic shots you hit in a game of tennis are called groundstrokes. They can be hit from anywhere after the ball has bounced, but they are most often played from near the baseline. There are two types of groundstrokes: forehand and backhand. A backhand can be played one- or two-handed.

① **Prepare to hit a forehand by turning your body, with your shoulders pointing into the court. Keep the racket arm alongside and away from the body.**

Turn your whole body

Turn your foot to the side to create an open stance

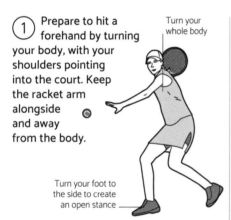

GRIP
Your grip determines how you strike the ball. Forehand grip positions include the Western and Semi-western. Western puts more topspin on the ball, while the Semi-western adds power.

Thumb

Pad of little finger

WESTERN

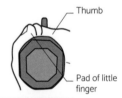

Thumb

Pad of little finger

SEMI-WESTERN

② **Swing your racket arm forward to play the ball. Turn your hips and shoulders to generate power in your stroke and hit through the ball.**

Rotate your shoulders to generate power

Push off through your foot as you make contact with the ball

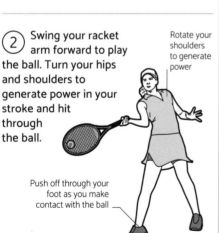

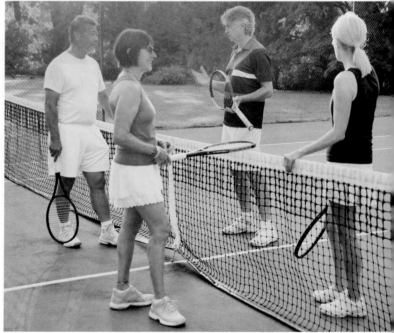

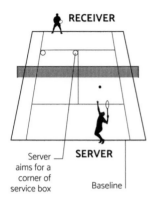

RECEIVER

Server aims for a corner of service box

SERVER

Baseline

CROSS-COURT

The server and receiver stand at opposite sides of the center service line. Serving well is not just about hitting a fast serve; the server must vary the placement of the ball to keep it out of the receiver's reach.

The fastest servers in men's tennis hit serves of over 150 mph (240 kph) in tournaments

SOCIAL BENEFITS

Tennis may be a competitive sport, but it can also be a relaxing social activity. Try a game of doubles or join a tennis club to play with people of similar ability.

EXERCISE 2 | ACING IT

Each point in a tennis match is begun with a serve. Most beginners start by serving underarm (hitting a forehand), but the ability to hit an accurate and powerful first serve that prevents an opponent from returning the ball is a big advantage.

(1) Throw the ball high in front of you with your free hand. Bend your knees as you throw the ball.

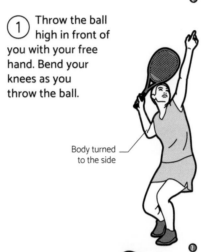

Body turned to the side

(2) Move your racket hand back behind you and bend your elbow. Push off with your legs as you start to swing your racket upward.

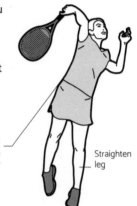

Turn body toward court to generate extra power

Straighten leg

(3) Swing your racket up, aiming to make contact with the ball before the ball starts falling fast. Aim to hit the ball with the middle of the racket head.

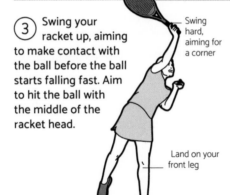

Swing hard, aiming for a corner

Land on your front leg

(4) Follow through with your swing, but try to keep your eye on the ball and prepare for a possible return of serve.

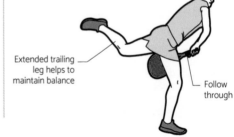

Extended trailing leg helps to maintain balance

Follow through

TAKE IT FURTHER

You can join a tennis league if you want to explore the competitive side of tennis further. Or there are many other racket sports to try, for example, squash and badminton, each with different challenges.

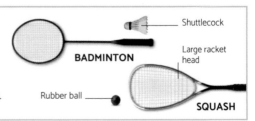

Shuttlecock

BADMINTON

Large racket head

Rubber ball

SQUASH

TRY GOLF

Hitting a golf ball straight and accurately over great distances requires excellent control over every joint in the body. Golf is a good way to get some gentle exercise and fresh air, but it also has a strong social side and provides for some healthy competition.

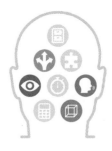

THINKING SKILLS

Improves focus and concentration

•

Develops spatial and navigation skills

•

Good for social interaction

EXERCISE 1 | GET A GRIP

One key to playing golf is knowing how to hold a club. A good grip allows you to hinge your wrists easily, meaning your clubhead will move fast as you swing. If you're gripping it right, your hands and forearms will naturally "waggle" the club.

(1) Start by feeding the handle into your left hand. The club falls into the fingers diagonally.

(2) The last three fingers squeeze the grip. The fingertips just touch the pad at the thumb's base.

(3) Introduce the right hand so that the left and right hands complement each other.

(4) Close the right hand. The left thumb sits under the fleshy pad at the base of the right thumb.

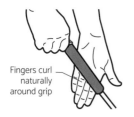

Fingers curl naturally around grip

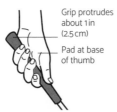

Grip protrudes about 1in (2.5 cm)

Pad at base of thumb

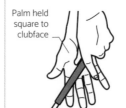

Palm held square to clubface

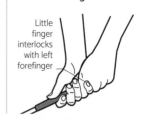

Little finger interlocks with left forefinger

EXERCISE 2 | TAKE A SWING

Hitting a golf ball a long way depends much more on timing and technique than on muscle power. Developing a good swing requires practice and attention to detail.

(3) Hinge your wrists to load up the swing, ready to unwind it on the downswing. Try a three-quarter swing before attempting a full swing.

(1) Bend from your hips, keeping a good flex in your knees. With arms hanging freely, your hands are beneath your chin.

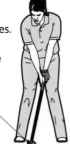

Before starting the swing, "address" the ball (ground the clubhead just behind it)

(2) As you begin your backswing, your upper body rotates, but your hips and knees resist this turning.

Club begins backswing

Arms and shoulders move as a triangle

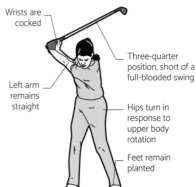

Wrists are cocked

Left arm remains straight

Three-quarter position, short of a full-blooded swing

Hips turn in response to upper body rotation

Feet remain planted

EXERCISE 3 |
GOLF CRAZY

Unless you can get a hole-in-one off every tee, you are going to need putting skills to get the ball into the hole. You can practice putting in the yard or even on the living room carpet, but you can make it more challenging by building your own miniature golf course. No need to buy equipment—just see what you can find to make a few obstacles.

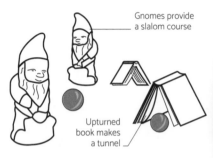

Gnomes provide a slalom course

Upturned book makes a tunnel

MINI PUTTING
For putting practice, buckets, guttering, tin cans, or even gnomes, are just some of the objects that can be put to use.

TAKE IT FURTHER

Take lessons at a local club to get advice on technique and get off to a flying start. Use a driving range or putting green if you can't get to a club. Golf equipment can be expensive, so look for secondhand sets. You can even experiment with foot golf or disk golf, or try swinging a croquet mallet instead of a golf club.

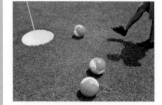

FOOT GOLF

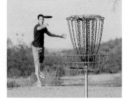

DISK GOLF

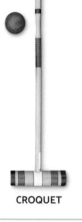

CROQUET

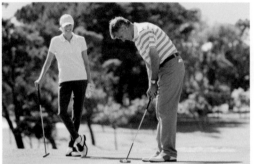

PLAYING PARTNER

A full-length, 18-hole golf course is typically 6,000–7,000 yards (5.5–6.5 km) long, and a round can take all morning or all afternoon. There is plenty of time to chat with your playing companions or opponents.

---

(4) Unwind your swing from the ankles upward. As your upper body shifts back toward the ball, your hands should fall into a hitting position. Keep your wrists hinged, loaded with energy.

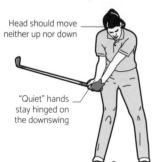

Head should move neither up nor down

"Quiet" hands stay hinged on the downswing

(5) Shortly before impact, unhinge your wrists to deliver a final burst of speed. You should feel the centrifugal force of the accelerating clubhead.

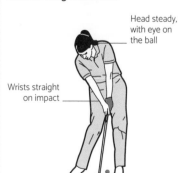

Head steady, with eye on the ball

Wrists straight on impact

(6) The momentum of your body continues your rotation into the follow-through. You should be able to hold this balanced position for a few seconds.

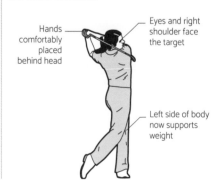

Hands comfortably placed behind head

Eyes and right shoulder face the target

Left side of body now supports weight

TRY SWIMMING

Swimming is an all-body exercise that increases blood flow, helping heart health and pumping oxygen and nutrients to the brain. Swimming also helps relax the body and mind.

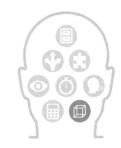

THINKING SKILLS

Reduces stress
•
Improves blood flow
•
Improves physical coordination

CHALLENGE 1 | BREASTSTROKE

One of the easiest swimming strokes, breaststroke is great for both competitive and leisurely swimming. Breathe in when your head comes up out of the water, or keep your head out of the water the whole time, if you prefer.

① With your legs and arms out straight, turn your palms outward. Pull the water out and around, bringing your elbows in to your sides.

Angle your arms down slightly for a stronger pull

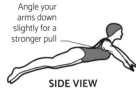

SIDE VIEW

Gradually bend your elbows and bring them back in to your sides

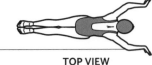

TOP VIEW

② Bring your palms together in front of your chest with your elbows bent, lifting your head and shoulders up and out of the water.

Tuck your elbows into your sides

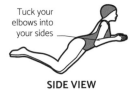

SIDE VIEW

Legs start getting ready to kick as your shoulders come up

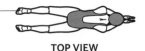

TOP VIEW

③ Push your arms out in front of you with your palms together—at the same time, bend your knees and kick out and together like a frog.

Bring your heels toward your bottom

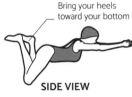

SIDE VIEW

When you kick out, push the water away with the inside edges and soles of your feet

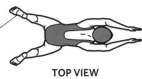

TOP VIEW

OUTDOOR SWIMMING
Open water swimming—in aquatic landscape features, such as a lake or the sea—improves blood circulation and can boost your immune system. Make sure to swim with an experienced companion the first few times.

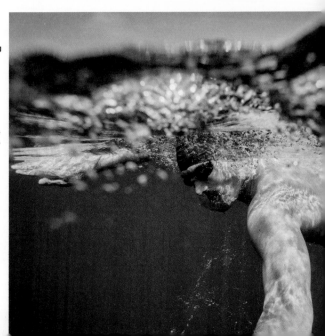

CHALLENGE 2 | **FRONT CRAWL**

The fastest swimming stroke, front crawl takes a little more energy. It is usually used in competitive freestyle races. Breathe when you need to by turning your head to the side as you bring your arm over your head.

(1) Keep one arm out in front of you and bring the other hand down to scoop the water down and underneath your body. Kick with your legs all the time.

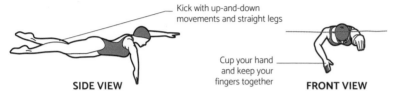

Kick with up-and-down movements and straight legs

Cup your hand and keep your fingers together

SIDE VIEW

FRONT VIEW

(2) Keep pushing the water until your hand has come up to your hip. Bring your hand out of the water behind you, and then up and over your head.

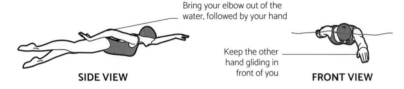

Bring your elbow out of the water, followed by your hand

Keep the other hand gliding in front of you

SIDE VIEW

FRONT VIEW

(3) Bring your hand down into the water, fingertips first, ahead of your head. Let this arm now glide in front of you as the other arm starts the movements you just did.

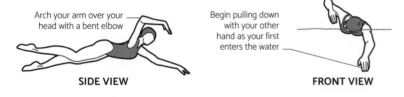

Arch your arm over your head with a bent elbow

Begin pulling down with your other hand as your first enters the water

SIDE VIEW

FRONT VIEW

People will be advised to swim in a circular path up and down the lane

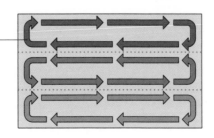

LANE SWIMMING
At "lane swim" sessions, the pool will be split up and signs will usually advise of the speed in each lane, so that people with the same swimming speed will be together.

TAKE IT FURTHER

Focus on strengthening particular body areas by using some simple equipment. Hold a pull buoy between your thighs while you swim, to help build your upper body strength. You could hold a kickboard out in front of you with your hands to focus on exercising your legs. Try swim fins on your feet to help improve your propulsive power.

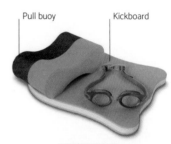

Pull buoy   Kickboard

EQUIPMENT

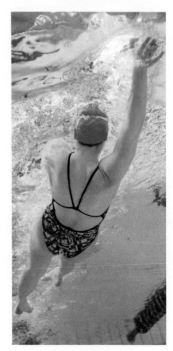

BACKSTROKE

TRY YOGA

Yoga is good for mind and body and can be performed by any age group. You can do it at home, but it is best to start with classes so that you can be instructed how to make the poses comfortably and find the poses that are most suitable for you.

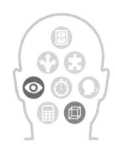

THINKING SKILLS

Focuses on mind and body as one

Improves flexibility and posture

Relieves stress

Relaxing and meditative

Workout for all muscle groups

EXERCISE 1 | ADOPT THE POSITION

A yoga session consists of a number of poses, or asanas, that complement each other to work key areas of the body. Always do some warm-up stretches first. Change it up, though–do not settle into a routine. Introduce new pose sequences every day or focus on something specific, such as leg muscles, core strength, or breathing. Do this for a week or more, then move onto something new.

DOWNWARD-FACING DOG
Start this pose by placing your hands and knees onto the ground. Then lift both knees off the ground and push your hips up and backward, keeping your arms and legs straight.

Try to keep your shoulders open and relaxed

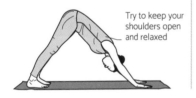

COBRA
Lie on your front, keeping your feet together and your legs straight. On an inhalation, lift your head and arch your back. Do not try to lift more than is comfortable.

Draw your shoulder blades back

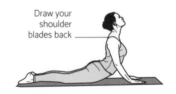

BRIDGE
Start on your back, with your feet a hip-width apart and your knees bent. Raise your hips and place your hands on your back, keeping your neck, head, and shoulders on the floor.

Place your hands on your back, not your hips.

Keep your feet flat on the floor

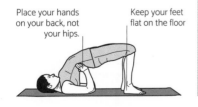

TREE
Start with both feet together, then lift one knee and bring your raised foot to the thigh of your standing leg. If that is comfortable and stable, raise your hands above your head.

Push down into your mat for stability

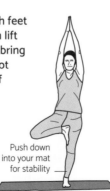

IMPROVING ALIGNMENT
Yoga is great for increasing flexibility, and a class is a fun, social way to learn poses and how to modify them to suit your ability.

EXERCISE 2 | IMPROVE YOUR CONCENTRATION WITH YOGA

Everyday life is full of distractions that can seriously disrupt attempts to concentrate on a specific project. Yoga can help improve your focus by helping you to relax. Regularly practicing certain poses, such as the lotus, corpse, tree, and mountain asanas, and deep breathing techniques will help you feel mentally refreshed.

1. Sit with a straight back. Cross your legs and find a posture that is comfortable for you.

2. Place your hands with palms facing upward on top of your knees.

3. Focus on your breathing. Take deep, slow breaths. Random thoughts may come to you—acknowledge them and let them go. To help you focus, try counting backward from 200.

4. Start with 10 minutes and gradually work your way up to longer periods. With regular practice, you will be able to use your breathing to regain your focus even when surrounded by distractions.

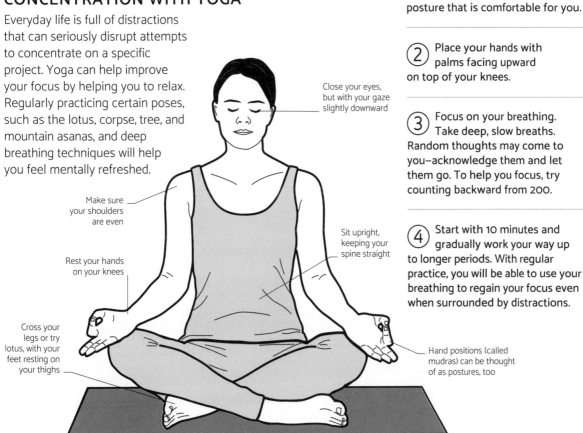

Close your eyes, but with your gaze slightly downward

Make sure your shoulders are even

Rest your hands on your knees

Cross your legs or try lotus, with your feet resting on your thighs

Sit upright, keeping your spine straight

Hand positions (called mudras) can be thought of as postures, too

TAKE IT FURTHER

Try different forms of yoga to find one that suits you. Ashtanga, Iyengar, Kundalini, power, and restorative yoga are among several you could try, according to how active you want to be. There are also teachers who specialize in prenatal yoga practice. Or try related disciplines, such as Pilates (see p.169), or add weight training into your routine to strengthen key areas.

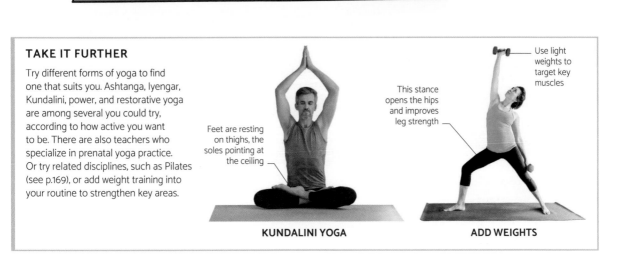

Feet are resting on thighs, the soles pointing at the ceiling

This stance opens the hips and improves leg strength

Use light weights to target key muscles

KUNDALINI YOGA

ADD WEIGHTS

TRY TAI CHI

Tai chi is an ancient Chinese martial art that can be practised by people with both full or limited mobility. This graceful art has been described as "moving meditation."

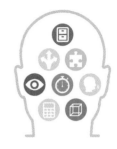

BENEFITS

Improves fitness levels

•

Reduces stress, anxiety, and depression

•

Improves spatial awareness

•

Boosts concentration

CHALLENGE 1 | TAKING A STANCE

There are many tai chi styles and forms (a form is a set of sequences), but each form begins in a normal upright stance. There should be no tension in the muscles. Next, try standing with your feet apart and your knees bent.

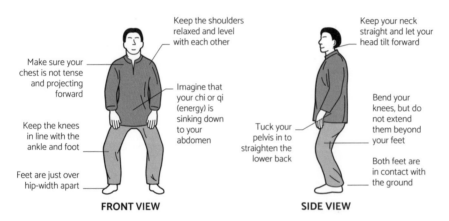

Keep the shoulders relaxed and level with each other

Make sure your chest is not tense and projecting forward

Imagine that your chi or qi (energy) is sinking down to your abdomen

Keep the knees in line with the ankle and foot

Feet are just over hip-width apart

FRONT VIEW

Keep your neck straight and let your head tilt forward

Tuck your pelvis in to straighten the lower back

Bend your knees, but do not extend them beyond your feet

Both feet are in contact with the ground

SIDE VIEW

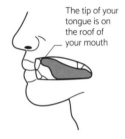

The tip of your tongue is on the roof of your mouth

BREATHING
Breathe in and out through your nose, and focus on keeping your breathing even.

CHALLENGE 2 | OPENING SEQUENCE

Some tai chi forms have more than 100 steps, but one of the most common forms for beginners has 24 steps. The opening sequence of this form is the transition from an upright stance with your feet together to a wider stance, and then a gentle upward and downward movement of the arms.

(1) **START UPRIGHT**
Stand comfortably, with your feet together and your arms hanging comfortably at your sides.

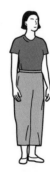

(2) **SHIFT WEIGHT**
Bend your knees and shift your weight into your right foot, but focus on not leaning over.

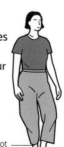

"Fill" your right foot with your weight

(3) **STEP OUT**
When all your weight is in your right leg, place your left foot about hip-width to the left.

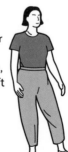

(4) **BALANCE**
Shift your weight into your left foot until your weight is spread equally. As you do this, turn your palms to face backward.

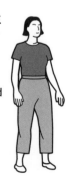

CHALLENGE 3 | STEPPING

Moving from one tai chi posture to another often requires the fluid transference of weight from one leg to another. When practising stepping, try to keep the movements even, and do not come to a complete stop at any part of a movement.

> **TAKE IT FURTHER**
> ● Find a beginner's class or a teacher who can help you learn a form. They will make sure your postures are correct and won't cause injury.
> ● Learn qigong, the practice of cultivating internal energy.

① START
Begin with your feet hip-width apart.

Keep your hands at your hips to ensure that you turn correctly

A grid helps you place your feet

② SHIFT YOUR WEIGHT
Move your weight into your left leg, but try to stay upright.

③ TURN YOUR HIPS
With the weight in your left leg, allow your hips to turn. Your right foot turns 45° to the side.

④ SHIFT AND STEP
Lower your right foot to the ground and shift your weight into it. This frees up your left leg for a forward step.

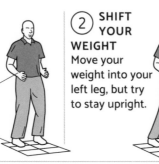

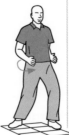

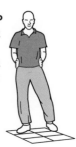

⑤ STEP
Each step you take is a controlled transference of your weight—gently place your left heel down first.

⑥ SHIFT WEIGHT FORWARD
Then shift your weight so that it is 70 percent in the front leg. Hips face forward.

⑦ WEIGHT BACK
Sink your weight into your back foot and turn your hips (and front foot) 45°.

⑧ SHIFT WEIGHT
Step forward with the back foot and transfer your weight. Your hips and front foot face forward.

⑤ LIFT ARMS
Raise your arms up to shoulder height, but stay relaxed.

Lead with the wrist and keep the elbows down

⑥ AT THE TOP
Straighten your wrists, with fingers pointing forward.

Take care not to raise your shoulders

⑧ ARMS DOWN
Leading with the wrist, lower your arms to your side.

Bend the wrists

⑨ FINISH AND BEGIN AGAIN
Arm movements are repeated three times.

Finish with your hands by your side

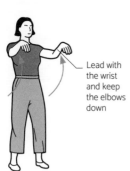

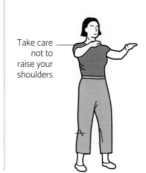

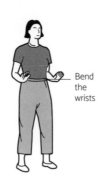

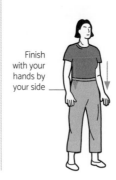

TRY DANCING

Thanks to a number of TV shows, ballroom and Latin dancing are becoming more popular than ever. Dancing is a great way to socialize and exercise your brain and body.

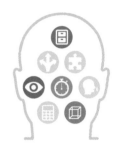

THINKING SKILLS

Improves physical coordination

•

Helps balance and spatial memory

•

Releases endorphins

EXERCISE 1 | SOCIAL FOXTROT

The social foxtrot is a simple ballroom dance that repeats a pattern of eight steps danced in a box shape. The steps are danced to a slow… slow… quick-quick timing, where the "slow" steps use two beats in the music and "quick" steps use one.

① LEADER'S STEPS
In ballroom dances, couples travel counterclockwise around the floor, with the person who is leading facing the outside of the ballroom. When you reach a corner, shorten or lengthen your stride slightly (keeping the same timing) as you turn.

② PARTNER'S STEPS
In Foxtrot, the partner's steps are very similar to the leader's steps. Why not take turns being the leader in different dances? When the leader takes a step forward, the partner takes a step backward.

TAKE IT FURTHER

You don't need a partner for line dancing, because everyone dances the same routine, with everyone facing in the same way. The routines use sequences of steps that are repeated. Although line dancing developed from country and western music, today it combines many different dance and music genres.

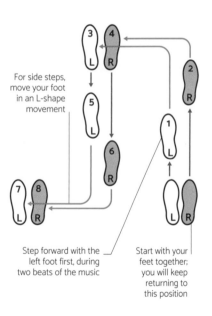

For side steps, move your foot in an L-shape movement

Step forward with the left foot first, during two beats of the music

Start with your feet together; you will keep returning to this position

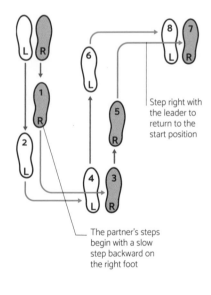

Step right with the leader to return to the start position

The partner's steps begin with a slow step backward on the right foot

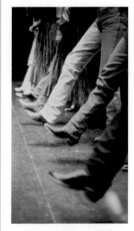

TRADITIONAL WEAR

KEY	→ Quick step (1 beat)	→ Slow step (2 beats)

EXERCISE 2 | CHA CHA CHA

The cha cha cha (sometimes just called the cha cha) is a fun Latin dance that originated in Cuba. In the basic routine below, each person in the partnership uses the same steps, but the leader starts from step 1 and the partner starts at step 6. So, when the leader steps forward (step 4), the partner will step backward (step 9). The rhythm of the sequence below is easiest to count as cha-cha-cha, ...2, ...3, cha-cha-cha, ...2, ...3.

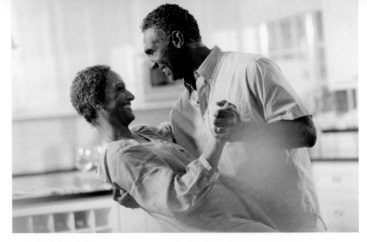

LEARN TOGETHER
Taking a friend or partner with you to a new class may help you to feel more confident–learning together might even make dancing more fun.

① Start with your feet together. Take a sidestep right, your first "cha."

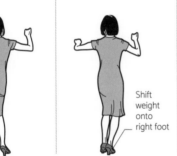

② Bring your left foot to your right foot, for the second "cha."

Shift weight onto right foot

③ Step right for the final "cha" of the "cha-cha-cha" rhythm steps.

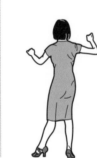

④ On the "...2" beat, step forward with your left foot.

Keep right foot's toes in place

⑤ Then, on the "...3" beat, shift your weight back onto your right foot.

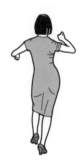

⑩ On the "...3" beat, shift your weight onto your front (left) foot.

From this position, start again from step 1

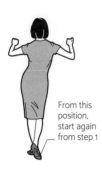

⑨ On the "...2" beat, step backward onto your right foot.

Keep left (front) foot in place

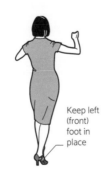

⑧ Step left for the final "cha" of the "cha-cha-cha" rhythm steps.

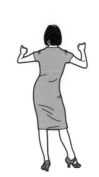

⑦ Bring your right foot to your left foot, for the second "cha."

Shift weight onto left foot

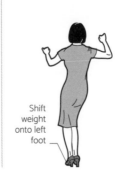

⑥ Bring back your left foot and sidestep to the left, for your next "cha."

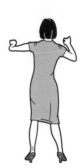

TRY STRENGTH TRAINING

Simple strength exercises and Pilates workouts can be done at home, and they help to keep both your mind and body strong. Even gentle exercise releases endorphins into the bloodstream.

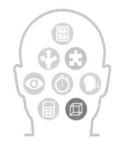

IMPROVING BODY STRENGTH

There are many strength workouts that you can do at home; try out a combination of the exercises below—aim for at least five steady repetitions of each one. Always begin with a 5–10-minute warm-up, such as walking on the spot.

SUPERMAN

(1) Get onto your hands and knees on a mat, keeping your back straight and stomach pulled in.

Place your hands shoulder-width apart

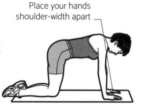

(2) Lift one arm up in front of you and lift the opposite leg out behind you; hold for a few seconds.

Do not twist your hips

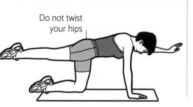

ROTATIONAL LUNGE STRETCH

Lunge your left leg forward. As you lower your body, twist your torso to the right. Repeat on the other side.

Bring your left arm across your body

Twist from your waist

Feel the stretch in the front of your right hip and your left buttock

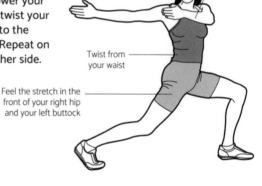

STANDING Y

(1) Stand with your feet hip-width apart. Hold a weight such as a dumbbell or bottle of water in each hand.

Keep back straight

Keep knees slightly bent

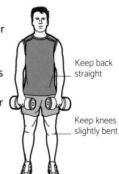

(2) Keeping your stomach tight, slowly lift the weights up, with each arm angled out at 45°.

Relax shoulders

Keep elbows slightly bent

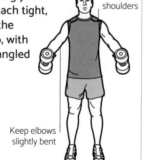

(3) Keeping your arms at 45°, raise the weights to shoulder height, then slowly lower.

Keep your core engaged

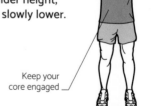

PILATES

Pilates is done either on a mat on the floor or on apparatus developed by Joseph Pilates. It aims to strengthen the body in an even way, with focus on your breathing and core strength. Practitioners say that regular Pilates can improve posture, muscle tone, and balance–and relieve stress and tension.

ONE LEG CIRCLE

(1) Lie down flat on a mat. Lift one leg up to the sky and point your toes.

(2) Direct your foot outward and then down slightly to draw small circles in the air.

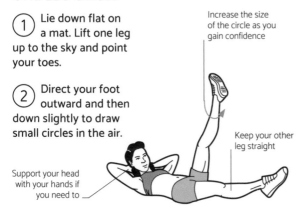

Increase the size of the circle as you gain confidence

Keep your other leg straight

Support your head with your hands if you need to

ROLLING LIKE A BALL

(1) Sit on a mat with your knees bent, holding your legs in to your body. Curve your back.

(2) Roll back onto your shoulders and then gently roll back up into a sitting position.

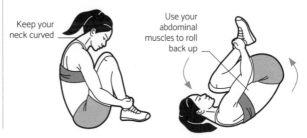

Keep your neck curved

Use your abdominal muscles to roll back up

TAKE IT FURTHER

Pilates can involve using special apparatus, such as a reformer (see below). You will need to attend a Pilates studio or class at your gym to try out these exercises, where a qualified Pilates instructor can help you learn how to get the most out of your Pilates workout. At the gym, you could also try your own workouts and make use of the gym's equipment. Be sure to ask a member of staff for advice and get the best workout for you.

The foot bar acts as a perch for feet or hands, and as a launchpad when using the carriage

The carriage can move along the frame while you are resting on it

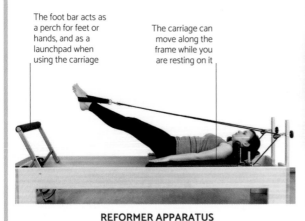

REFORMER APPARATUS

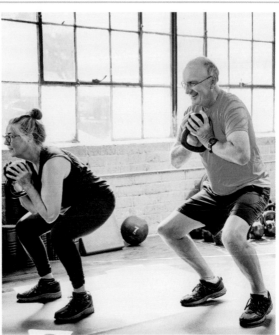

SQUATS WITH KETTLEBELL WEIGHTS

TRY A NEW LANGUAGE

You are never too old to learn a new language. To achieve conversational fluency you need only 2,000–3,000 words. You don't need to go this far, however, to get a mental workout. You can just dip in, learn a few words and phrases, and find out how a language works. Make a start with these.

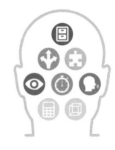

THINKING SKILLS

Exercises memory

•

Increases ability with words

•

Forces the brain to process unfamiliar information in novel ways

•

Builds connections between neurons and makes grey matter denser

EXERCISE 1 | BECOME A POLYGLOT

Try learning these words for household items in French, German, Spanish, Italian, and Dutch. Practice saying them for 10 minutes every day. Once you have mastered them, try learning them in another language. Mix it up by alternating between languages as you name the items.

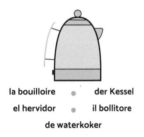

la bouilloire	•	der Kessel
el hervidor	•	il bollitore
de waterkoker		

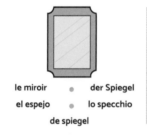

le miroir	•	der Spiegel
el espejo	•	lo specchio
de spiegel		

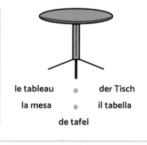

le tableau	•	der Tisch
la mesa	•	il tabella
de tafel		

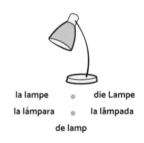

la lampe	•	die Lampe
la lámpara	•	la lâmpada
de lamp		

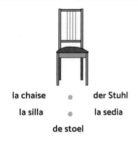

la chaise	•	der Stuhl
la silla	•	la sedia
de stoel		

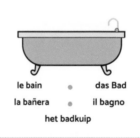

le bain	•	das Bad
la bañera	•	il bagno
het badkuip		

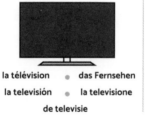

la télévision	•	das Fernsehen
la televisión	•	la televisione
de televisie		

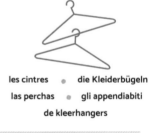

les cintres	•	die Kleiderbügeln
las perchas	•	gli appendiabiti
de kleerhangers		

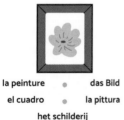

la peinture	•	das Bild
el cuadro	•	la pittura
het schilderij		

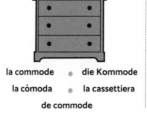

la commode	•	die Kommode
la cómoda	•	la cassettiera
de commode		

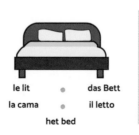

le lit	•	das Bett
la cama	•	il letto
het bed		

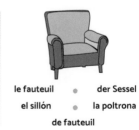

le fauteuil	•	der Sessel
el sillón	•	la poltrona
de fauteuil		

EXERCISE 2 | COUNT ON IT

Numbers are a vital part of speaking a language. Most languages have specific names for the first 10 or 20 numbers, and name higher numbers using a combination of these. For example, the number 23 is built from words for "20" and "three"–twenty-three (English), veintitrés (Spanish), vingt-trois (French), and dreiundzwanzig (three-and-twenty, German). This can result in long, compound words as the numbers get bigger, especially as they reach the thousands.

2,345

English–two thousand, three hundred and forty-five
Italian–duemilatrecentoquarantacinque
German–zweitausenddreihundertfünfundvierzig
Swedish–tvåtusentrehundrafyrtiofem

1 These are the words for numbers up to 1,000 in five languages. Notice how they build on earlier numbers as they get bigger.

	0	1	2	3	4	5	6	7	8	9
Spanish	cero	uno	dos	tres	cuatro	cinco	seis	siete	ocho	nueve
French	zéro	un	deux	trois	quatre	cinq	six	sept	huit	neuf
Italian	zero	uno	duo	tre	quattro	cinque	sei	sette	otto	nove
German	null	ein	zwei	drei	vier	fünf	sechs	sieben	acht	neun
Swedish	noll	ett	två	tre	fyra	fem	sex	sju	åtta	nio

	10	11	12	13	14	15	16	17	18	19
Spanish	diez	once	doce	trece	catorce	quince	dieciséis	diecisiete	dieciocho	diecinueve
French	dix	onze	douze	treize	quatorze	quinze	seize	dix-sept	dix-huit	dix-neuf
Italian	dieci	undici	dodici	tredici	quattordici	quindici	sedici	diciassette	diciotto	diciannove
German	zehn	elf	zwölf	dreizehn	vierzehn	fünfzehn	sechszehn	siebzehn	achtzehn	neunzehn
Swedish	tio	elva	tolv	tretton	fjorton	femton	sexton	sjutton	arton	nitton

	20	30	40	50	60	70	80	90	100	1,000
Spanish	veinte	treinta	cuarenta	cincuenta	sesenta	setenta	ochenta	noventa	cien	mil
French	vingt	trente	quarante	cinquante	soixante	soixante-dix	quatre-vingt	quatre-vingt-dix	cent	mille
Italian	venti	trente	quaranta	cinquanta	sessanta	settanta	ottanta	novanta	cento	mille
German	zwanzig	dreizig	vierzig	fünfzig	sechszig	siebzig	achtzig	neunzig	hundert	tausend
Swedish	tjugo	trettio	fyrtio	femtio	sextio	sjuttio	åttio	nittio	hundra	tusen

2 Use the patterns in the names of numbers you see above to attempt these complex numbers. Follow the examples given at the beginning of the exercise for adding numbers in the tens, hundreds, and thousands.

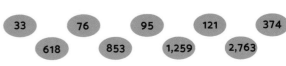

33   76   95   121   374
618   853   1,259   2,763

✦ Answers on page 187

EXERCISE 3 | WHAT'S THE TIME?

As in counting, speakers of different languages often have varying ways of expressing themselves when telling the time. Some put the minutes first, others the hours. In English, 1:30 is "one thirty," but in German, it is "halb-zwei" (half before two). In French, 3:40 is "trois heures moins vingt" (three hours, less twenty), and 1:20 in Arabic, is "waahda wi tilt" (one and a third). Many countries also use the 24-hour clock for times after noon. Can you remember how to tell these time in French, German, and Spanish?

quatorze heures quinze
vierzehn Uhr fünfzehn
las catorce quince

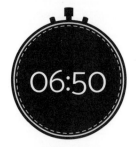

sept heures moins dix
zehn vor sieben
las seis cincuenta

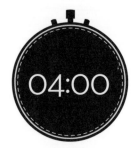

quatre heures
vier Uhr
las cuatro

vingt-et-une heures vingt-cinq
einundzwanzig Uhr fünfundzwanzig
las veintiuno veinticinco

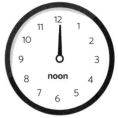

midi
Mittag
mediodía

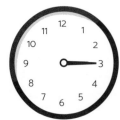

trois heures et quart
Viertel nach drei
las tres y cuarto

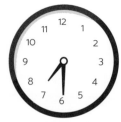

sept heures et demie
halb-acht
las siete y media

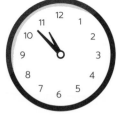

onze heures moins huit
acht vor elf
las once menos ocho

minuit
Mitternach
medianoche

treize heures quinze
dreizehn Uhr fünfzehn
las trece quince

dix-huit heures quarante-cinq
Viertel vor neunzehn
las dieciocho cuarenta y cinco

vingt-trois heures trente-six
vierundzwanzig vor Mitternach
las veintitrés treinta y seis

EXERCISE 4 | BE FLASH

Flash cards are a useful way to learn new words. You can use a set of children's flash cards for everyday items, or make your own. Put a picture on one side and the word for it on the back. That way, you can use both sides to translate both pictures and words. These use English, French, German, and Spanish.

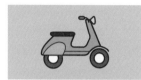

scooter
le scooter
der Motorroller
el scooter

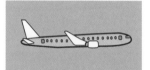

airplane
l'avion
das Flugzeug
el avión

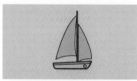

yacht
le yacht
die Yacht
el yate

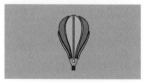

hot-air balloon
la montgolfière
der Heißluftballon
el globo aerostático

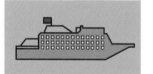

ship
le bateau
das Schiff
el barco

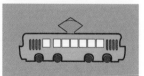

trolley
le tram
die Straßenbahn
el tranvía

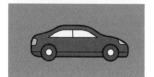

car
l'auto
das Auto
el coche

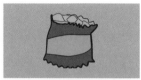

potato chips
les chips
die Kartoffelchips
las patatas fritas

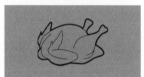

chicken
le poulet
das Huhn
el pollo

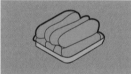

sausages
les saucissons
die Würstchen
las salchichas

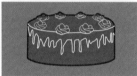

cake
le gâteaux
der Kuchen
la tarta

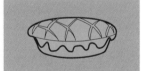

pie
la tarte
die Torte
el pastel

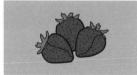

strawberries
les fraises
die Erdbeeren
las fresas

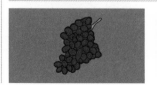

grapes
les raisins
die Trauben
las uvas

EXERCISE 5 | QUESTIONS, QUESTIONS, QUESTIONS

Meeting a foreign person or traveling to a new country involves questions. You may be the person asking the question or you may be being asked and have to reply. It also pays to learn basic greetings, and manners are always appreciated. Here are some common phrases for you to try.

	FRENCH	GERMAN	SPANISH
How are you? I'm fine, thanks.	Comment allez-vous? Je vais bien, merci.	Wie geht es Ihnen? Es geht mir gut, danke.	¿Cómo está? Estoy bien, gracias.
Pleased to meet you	Enchanté	Angenehm	Encantado de conocerle
You're welcome!	De rien	Bitte schön/Bitte sehr	De nada
I'm sorry/ excuse me	Pardon/Excusez-moi	Es tut mir leid/ Entschuldigung	Lo siento/Perdone
My name is… / What is your name?	Je m'appelle… /Comment appellez vous?	Ich heiße… / Wie heißen Sie?	Me llamo… /¿Cómo se llama?
Where do you live/come from?	Où habitez-vous/Vous êtes d'où?	Wo wohnen Sie?/Wo kommen Sie her?	¿De dónde es usted?
What time is it?	Quelle heure est-il?	Wie spät ist es?	¿Qué hora es?
What do you do?	Quel est votre métier?	Was ist Ihre Aufgabe?	¿En qué trabaja?
Hello/goodbye	Bonjour/Au revoir	Hallo/Auf Wiedersehen	Hola/Adiós
Please/thank you	S'il vous plaît/Merci	Bitte/Danke	Por favor/Gracias
Good morning/ afternoon	Bonjour/Bonjour	Guten Morgen/Guten Tag	Buenos días/Buenas tardes
I don't understand	Je ne comprends pas	Ich verstehe nicht	No entiendo

head
la tête
der Kopf
la cabeza

hair
les cheveux,
das Haar
el pelo

eye
l'oeil
das Auge
el ojo

nose
le nez
die Nase
la nariz

ear
l'oreille
das Ohr
la oreja

mouth
la bouche
der Mund
la boca

neck
le cou
der Hals
el cuello

chest
la poitrine
die Brust
el pecho

abdomen
le ventre
der Bauch
el abdomen

arm
le bras
der Arm
el brazo

waist
la taille
die Taille
la cintura

hand
la main
die Hand
la mano

finger
le doigt
der Finger
el dedo

knee
le genou
das Knie
la rodilla

leg
la jambe
das Bein
la pierna

foot
le pied
der Fuß
el pie

EXERCISE 6 | BODY PARTS

Knowing the parts of the body in another language is useful in the event of becoming sick or having an accident. Try these in French, German, and Spanish.

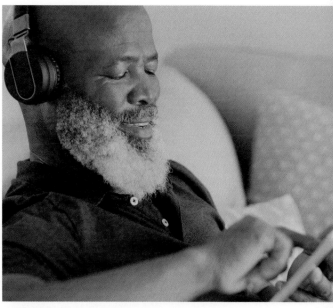

LISTEN IN
Audioguides and apps can walk you through the first steps of learning a language, and can give you essential experience of listening to the sound of native speakers.

Practice vocabulary whenever you can, even if it is for just a few minutes. The best time to learn is just before you go to sleep, as this helps to lay down memories

EXERCISE 7 | **HANGMAN**

Hangman is a game that is good for revising vocabulary and practicing the alphabet of another language. You can use a preselected list of words or use those from earlier exercises. Participants each say a letter and if it isn't in the word, the hangman starts to be drawn.

(1) One player thinks of a word and draws a series of dashes representing letters in the word.

(2) Other players take turns guessing the letters.

(3) The first player writes any correct letters in their right place on top of the dashes.

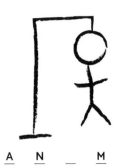

H A N _ M A N

(4) For each incorrect letter, the first player draws one part of the hangman's scaffold and body.

(5) If the scaffold and figure are completed before the word is guessed, the first player wins.

(6) If another player says the word before being hanged, they win.

EXERCISE 8 | **THE PICNIC GAME**

Prepare an imaginary picnic. Each player takes a turn saying what they will contribute: "I'm going on a picnic and I'm bringing…." You can use the items below and those in Exercise 4 as ideas for what to take. You can make it more taxing by repeating the previous players' items before naming a new object. This is how you would start the game in these languages:

: **To test your memory, you could list all the previous foods before naming a new one**

French–"Je vais faire un pique-nique et j'apporte…"

German–"Ich gehe zu einem Picknick und bringe…"

Spanish–"Voy a ir a un picnic y voy a llevar…"

les oranges
die Orangen
las naranjas

le pain
das Brot
el pan

le yaourt
der Joghurt
el yogurt

les pommes
die Äpfel
las manzanas

les sandwiches
die Sandwiches
los sándwiches

le jus d'orange
der Orangensaft
el zumo de naranja

les bananes
die Bananen
los plátanos

le fromage
der Käse
el queso

l'eau
das Wasser
el agua

les mangues
die Mangos
los mangos

le pastèque
die Wassermelone
la sandía

la limonade
die Limonade
la limonade

TAKE IT FURTHER

DIFFERENT WRITING SYSTEMS

You may want to learn a language that uses a different writing system–this introduces a whole extra dimension to your mental workout.

> **Avoid using Roman script for a language that uses another writing system–it will give you a bad accent!**

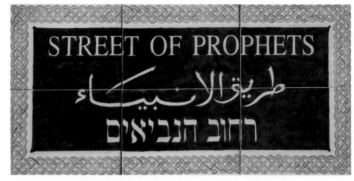

STREET SIGN IN ENGLISH, ARABIC, AND HEBREW

LISTEN VERY CAREFULLY

To have a conversation in another language you need to develop an ear for how it is spoken. Take any opportunity to listen to native speakers, whether in person or through various media. You can also join a conversation group.

Follow stories you know about on international news channels

Try watching foreign films with subtitles and then without subtitles to follow the dialogue

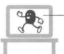
Watch children's programs for their simplicity of ideas and language

Find the foreign lyrics for a song you know and sing along to a backing track

TALKING TO COMPUTERS

The discipline of learning computer code is a little like learning a language, but you also have to train yourself to think like a computer. You must specify instructions precisely, covering all possibilities. Scratch is a visual coding language that is a great environment for learning the principles. Python is a more versatile, text-based language. It is made of recognizable words and characters, so it can be easily read and understood by humans.

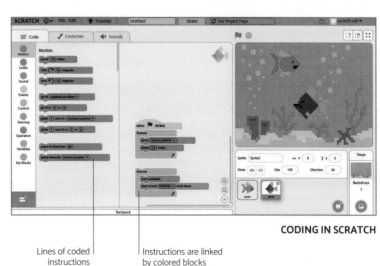

CODING IN SCRATCH

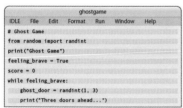

CODING IN PYTHON

Lines of coded instructions

Instructions are linked by colored blocks

TAKING UP THE CHALLENGE

It's one thing to know what to do to help keep your brain fit, and another to start doing it! The best way to get motivated is to join other people who share the same goals.

Seeing patterns where there are none, such as seeing a face in clouds, is known as pareidolia

GETTING STARTED

This book has hopefully sparked an interest in all sorts of new hobbies and activities for you to take up. Try out as many as you can, and continue building and strengthening your brain's networks—and have fun while you do it!

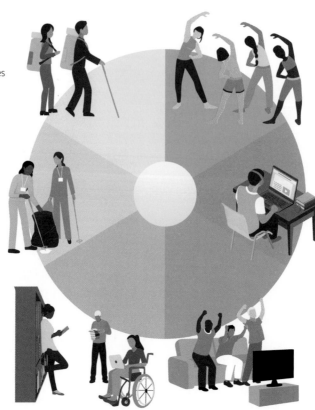

LOCAL GROUPS
Many things are best done in a group—check your local notice boards, newspapers, and websites for hobby groups or you could even start up your own.

CLUBS
Nearly every town and city has choirs, associations, and sports clubs. Look for notices in your leisure center or on social media to enjoy sports and activities with others.

VOLUNTEERING
However you dedicate your time, volunteering brings a double reward—take on a new challenge and also get the "feel-good" factor of making a difference.

CLASSES
Have you ever said "I wish I could..."? Never say it again—learn to do it! Find a local teacher, class, or just get a good book and start teaching yourself.

BOOKS
Join a book club to widen and deepen your reading through discussing books with others or pick up a nonfiction book and learn about a new subject.

MOVIES AND TV
Use a streaming service or Smart TV to watch some new movies or programs with friends, and discuss them afterward. Why not try a film in a different language?

USEFUL RESOURCES

HEALTH RESOURCES

Alzheimer's Association
Find out about Alzheimer's and dementia.
www.alz.org/

ChooseMyPlate (USDA)
A guide to eating balanced and healthy meals.
www.choosemyplate.gov/

Dementia Society of America
Support, information, and advice on dementia and Alzheimer's.
www.dementiasociety.org/

FindTreatment.gov
Advice and support on mental health and substance abuse.
www.findtreatment.gov/

Silver Sneakers
Find free local fitness classes, live online classes and workshops, and on-demand workouts.
www.silversneakers.com/

Verywell Fit
Get started on fitness with a 6-week beginner program.
www.verywellfit.com/six-weeks-fitness-absolute-beginners

OTHER RESOURCES

Chess Federation of Canada
Find chess leagues and clubs across Canada.
www.chess.ca/en/

Duolingo
Learn a new language for free through the website or app.
www.duolingo.com

Experience Corps
This volunteer opportunity links older tutors with young people in need of educational support.
www.aarp.org/experience-corps/

Move United
Learn about adaptive sports and local opportunities.
www.moveunitedsport.org/sports/adaptive-sports/

Parkrun
Free social 5K events at parks to walk, jog, or run: also includes volunteering opportunities.
www.parkrun.us/

USA Pickleball
A fun, social racket sport that can be played indoors or outdoors.
usapickleball.org/what-is-pickleball/

US Chess Federation
Find chess leagues and clubs across the United States.
new.uschess.org/

VolunteerMatch
Discover volunteering opportunities near you.
www.volunteermatch.org/

DK BOOKS

DK publishes beginner's guides to most of the activities featured in *The Brain Fitness Book*.

MUSIC AND ART
Artist's Drawing Techniques
Complete Pottery Techniques
Drawing Workshop
How to Draw
The Complete Guitar Manual

CRAFTS AND HOBBIES
Beginner Gardening Step by Step
Creative Paper Crafts
Crochet
Crochet Step by Step
How to Garden
How to Play Chess
Knit Step by Step
Knots: the Complete Visual Guide
The Knitting Book

NATURE
The Practical Astronomer
What's That Bird?
What's That Flower?
What's That Tree?

SPORTS AND FITNESS
15-Minute Pilates
The Complete Golf Manual
The Science of Strength Training
Yoga for Everyone

LANGUAGES
DK offers many useful guides and resources for learning a new language, including:

15-Minute Guides in: Arabic, French, German, Italian, Japanese, Chinese, and Spanish.

Complete Language Packs in: French, Italian, Chinese, and Spanish.

ANSWERS

CHAPTER 3

60–61 ABILITY WITH WORDS

1. ZIGZAG

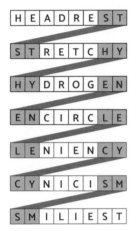

2. WORD CHAINS

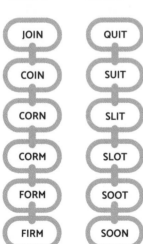

WORD CHAIN 1

WORD CHAIN 2

3. SHIFTED LETTERS
Each letter has been shifted by 13 places through the alphabet. The birds are: robin, swan, duck, jay, and parrot.

4. PATHFINDER
DRESSER, ARMCHAIR, FUTON, LAMP, MIRROR, WARDROBE, CUPBOARD, FOOTSTOOL, TABLE, SOFA

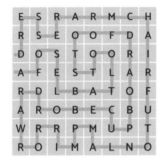

5. LETTER SOUP
The colors are brown, green, indigo, magenta, and orange.

6. WORD CIRCLE
The word that uses all of the letters is "discovery." Other words to be found include cove, cover, covers, coves, covey, coveys, discover, dive, diver, divers, dives, divorce, divorces, dove, doves, drive, drives, drove, droves, ivory, ivy, over, overs, rev, revs, rive, rives, servo, very, vice, viceroy, viceroys, vices, video, videos, vie, vied, vies, vireo, vireos, visor, voice, voiced, voices, void, and voids.

7. FIVE FOR FIVE
Words to be found include baler, batch, beech, belch, bream, dater, deter, dream, drear, haler, hatch, and hater.

62–65 ABILITY WITH NUMBERS

1. NUMBER DARTS
$60 = 15 + 14 + 31$
$70 = 27 + 20 + 23$
$85 = 15 + 30 + 40$

2. CIRCLE NUMBERS

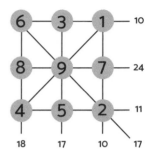

3. AGES AND AGES
Ali is 4 years old, Billi is 18 years old, and Charli is 12 years old.

4. BRAIN CHAINS

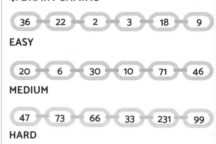

EASY

MEDIUM

HARD

5. A QUESTION OF LEGS
There are 15 goats. These 15 goats have 60 legs, leaving 16 geese legs to be attached to 8 geese. 15 goats and 8 geese together make 23 animals overall.

6. CUBIC COUNTING
There are 29 cubes.

7. MINI KROPKI

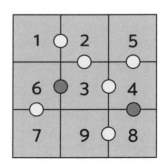

8. FLOATING NUMBERS

33 = 16 + 17
44 = 13 + 15 + 16
66 = 9 + 15 + 17 + 25

9. PROGENITORIAL PROBLEM

Mrs. A has 24 granddaughters (and 40 grandchildren overall). She has 6 sons and 3 daughters–who, of course, are the sisters to each brother. Mrs. A's 3 daughters have 2 sons each (for a total of 6 grandsons) and 3 daughters each (for a total of 9 granddaughters). All but one of Mrs. A's sons–that is, 5 of them–has 3 daughters each (for a total of 15 granddaughters) and 2 sons each (for a total of 10 grandsons). Mrs. A's other son has no children.

10. ARITHMETIC SQUARE

9	x	7	÷	3	=	21
x		+		x		
8	x	6	-	5	=	43
+		-		x		
2	+	4	+	1	=	7
=		=		=		
74		9		15		

11. A QUESTION OF SPEED

The boat, at an average of 27 mph. The car travels at 24 mph and the train at 26 mph.

12. GRAPE EXPECTATIONS

Each grape costs 5¢. There are 40 grapes in the bag to begin with, so when you eat half you leave 20. Your friend eats a fifth of 20 grapes–that is, 4 grapes–leaving 16. You then eat 4 more grapes each, for a total of 8 more, leaving 8 grapes. So if grapes cost $2 for 40 grapes, then one grape costs 200¢ ÷ 40, which is 5¢.

13. BAKERY DECISION

152 g. Each bagel weighs 40 g, and each doughnut weighs 56 g.

14. PAINTING PROBLEM

24 hours. We can see that Mr. A works three times as fast as Miss B, since it would only take them 2 hours more (compared to the original total of 6 hours) to do all of Miss B's work, too. Given this fact, instead of 8 hours, it would have taken 3x8 = 24 hours for Miss B to paint the house.

15. BRAIN CHAINS

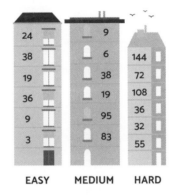

EASY   MEDIUM   HARD

16. HOUSE OF CARDS

9 layers. The lowest layer would have 10 cards in, the next layer up would have 4 flat cards, then 8 upright cards, then 3 flat cards, then 6 upright cards, then 2 flat cards, then 4 upright, then 1 flat, and finally 2 cards at the top, using 40 cards in total. This leaves only 12 cards, which is not enough for a flat layer of 5 plus an upright layer of 12 beneath.

66–69 PROBLEM-SOLVING

1. BIRTHDAY BOGGLER

Today is January 1. Two days ago, on December 30, he was 26. The next day, on December 31, he had his 27th birthday. Later this year, on December 31, he will turn 28. Then, next year, again on December 31, he will turn 29.

2. DRINK DIVISION

Pour into the 5-liter container, to leave 2 liters in the largest container. Next, pour the 5-liter container into the smallest one, leaving 3 liters in the midsized container. Pour the 2 liters from the small container into the largest one, so the large container now holds 4 liters. Now all you have to do is fill the 2-liter container again from the midsized container, and pour those 2 liters into the largest container.

3. PATH PROBLEM

The secret is to extend some of your lines far outside the boundaries of the grid of dots. For example:

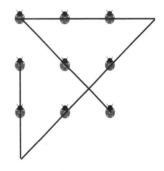

4. A QUESTION OF TRUTH

Person 4 could be telling the truth. Person 5 must be lying, because their statement would only be true if they were lying and so the statement itself would be false, resulting in an immediate contradiction. Meanwhile, persons 1 to 3 must be lying because in each case there needs to be at least one other person telling the truth, and yet all of the other statements would then contradict the exact number of people telling the truth. This leaves just person 4, whose statement could be true if they were themselves telling the truth.

5. CAKE CUTTING
Cut the cake horizontally across into two identical layers, then make two cuts at right angles through the center of the top of the cake, as shown:

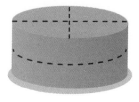

6. CARD CONFUSION
They should deal 25 cards into one pile, and leave the remaining 27 in the other. Then they should turn over the pile of 25 cards. To see why this works, imagine that there are "x" upside-down cards in the pile of 25. This means that there must be 25-x upside-down cards in the other pile (that is, all of those not in the first pile). But, when the first pile is turned the other way up, because there are 25 cards in that pile then the number of upside-down cards also becomes 25-x.

7. BOTTLING DILEMMA
Simply lay the bottle on its side. Because the bottle will then have perfect mirror symmetry from top to bottom, each half will hold the same volume and it will be easy to see by eye when half the volume of the bottle remains.

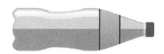

8. COIN CHALLENGE
Place three of the coins in a triangular arrangement, so each of the three coins touches both of the others in that triangle, and then place the fourth coin in the center on top of the triangle—so it touches all three of the coins beneath it.

9. CRATE EXPECTATIONS
First, put the smallest crate inside the largest crate, then place six apples into the smallest crate and six into the crate you have not yet used. Each crate will now have six apples inside it. This fulfills the requirements of the question, even if it hasn't magically created six extra apples!.

10. THE BACKWARD PANTS
Take the pants off and then put them back on backward, so your left leg goes in the right leg hole and vice-versa. Then it's an easy case of placing each hand just behind your back and into the opposite leg's pocket.

11. THE BURNING ROPES
Start by lighting one of the two ropes at both ends, and the other rope at just one end. When the rope lit at both ends has fully burned, 15 minutes will have passed, since—by being lit at both ends—it will have burned twice as quickly as if it had only been lit at one end. At this point, the other rope will still have 15 minutes' burning time left. Now light the second rope at its other end, which will in turn double the speed at which it burns—and therefore it will now take another $7\frac{1}{2}$ minutes to burn. This gives a total burn time of $22\frac{1}{2}$ minutes, as needed.

12. THE BOTTLE AND THE BEAN
Apply sufficient pressure to push the cork into the bottle, and then shake out the bean. As an alternative solution, you might also be able to drill out the center of the cork while pushing its fragments into the bottle, so as not to remove it from the bottle.

13. COUNTING CATS
Three cats: one white, one ginger, and one tortoiseshell.

14. CALENDAR SEARCH
Five. Each time you say a date, you are either correct or you can divide the month into two, and after dividing in two four times, you will have enough information to narrow it to a single date. The fifth date you say is therefore guaranteed to be correct. For this to work, your first guess should therefore be in the middle of the range of dates, 16, and then if the correct date is higher you then guess the center of the range between 16 and 31—that is, 24—or if it is lower, then you guess the center of the range between 1 and 16—that is, 8. This means you have a range of up to 16 dates after 1 guess, 8 dates after 2 guesses, 4 dates after 3 guesses, and 2 dates after 4 guesses. Because you are told "higher" or "lower," a range of 2 dates is sufficient to be certain of the answer.

15. STEEL AND WATER
You can use a magnet, since steel contains iron and is therefore magnetic. If the magnet is powerful enough, you won't need to touch the glass. Start at the bottom of the glass, near the screw, and move the magnet upward until the screw reaches the top of the glass and jumps across onto the magnet.

16. PIZZA PROBLEM

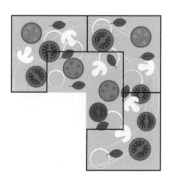

17. THE NON-LEAKY BUCKET
Spin the bucket up and over you in a loop. If you spin it at a suitable speed, then the centrifugal force that acts on the water will keep it in the bucket and prevent it from spilling out.

18. UNLIKELY AVERAGES

It depends on how you interpret the claim. If you interpret the average as referring to the mathematical mean of the height of all trees–that is, the most common meaning of "average" in a mathematical sense–then it could be true if the tallest 25 percent of trees were very much taller than the remaining shorter 75 percent of trees.

19. HOURGLASS DILEMMA

Turn both hourglasses over at the same time. When the 8-minute glass runs out, turn it over and start it again. At this point, there will still be 6 minutes of sand left to run in the 14-minute hourglass. When this hourglass runs out, turn the 8-minute glass over for a third time. Six minutes will have passed since its second turn, and so if turned at this point then there will be 6 minutes of sand left to run back through. When these 6 minutes of sand in the 8-minute glass have run all the way through, 20 minutes will have elapsed.

70-71 DECISION-MAKING

1. TRUTH AND LIES

B never lies. A must be lying because if they always lied then they couldn't admit it, so they must be the person who sometimes lies. B is telling the truth, because we know that A is the person who sometimes lies, and therefore–since B cannot by definition then be the liar–B must be the person who never lies.

2. THE BIASED COIN

Instead of calling "heads" or "tails," call "heads then tails" or "tails then heads" and flip the coin twice. If you get two heads or two tails then do two more flips. Otherwise, if you get two different results, then the bias of the coin won't have affected the result.

3. IF AND ONLY IF

Yes, they will. If they are the truth-teller then the second part of the statement is true, and therefore they will be going to the movies. If they are the liar, then the statement in the speech bubble is false and so they will not go to the movies if and only if they are the twin who tells the truth–but, since they aren't the truth-telling twin, then the "if and only" clause is not fulfilled and so the only condition on which they would not go to the movies does not occur, and so they are going to the movies. Therefore, no matter which twin you speak to, they will be going to the movies.

4. THE LABELED JARS

Taste the contents of the jar labeled "Sugar and Salt." You won't taste sugar and salt, since you know in advance that all of the labels are wrong. If you taste salt, you have found the salt. If you taste sugar, however, then the salt must be in the jar labeled "Sugar," since you know in advance it isn't in the "Salt" jar.

5. DIAMOND DECISION

You should switch cups. The cup originally chosen had a 1 in 3 chance of winning, and you can't change this. If you switch, however, then you know for certain you have a 1 in 2 chance of winning. This is a well-known probability paradox called the Monty Hall Problem.

6. DIE CHOICE

No. You have a less than even chance of winning, since the probability of you not rolling a six three times in a row is $5/6$ x $5/6$ x $5/6$ = 125/216, which is greater than half (108/216).

7. SQUASH

You should play Paul first, i.e., Paul, Peter, then Paul. Whomever you are playing, you must win the middle game to be able to win two games in a row, so it is best to play Peter for that game, since you are more likely to win–you then have two chances to win a game against the tougher player.

72-73 ATTENTION AND FOCUS

1. NUMBER SEARCH

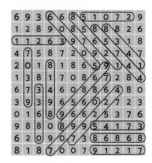

2. CIRCUIT BOARD

Piece 3.

3. ODD ONE OUT

Shape C, since it has only 5 sides, while the other three shapes all have 6 sides.

4. WARP MAZE

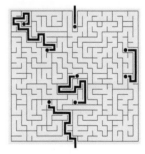

5. CUBE CONUNDRUM

Cube D.

6. TWISTING TOTAL

11 left turns:

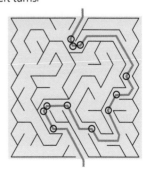

7. MISSING FACE Face D.

74–75 THINKING SPEED AND REACTION TIME

1. MISSING DOMINO
The only domino that cannot be formed is the 3-6 / 6-3 domino.

2. BRIDGE MAZE

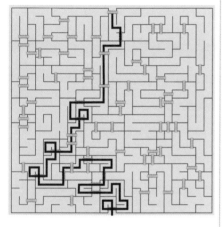

3. OUT OF SEQUENCE
D. The sequence, once D is restored, becomes Roman numerals in decreasing order of value, with M=1000, D=500, C=100, L=50, X=10, V=5, and I=1.

4. SUDOKU ERROR
The square marked with a star should be changed to a 5. Currently, it duplicates the three circled 2s.

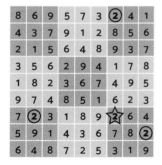

5. COUNTRY INTERSECTION
Rule A: Countries in which most people speak Spanish as a first language.
Rule B: Countries that are also islands.

6. SPOT THE DIFFERENCE

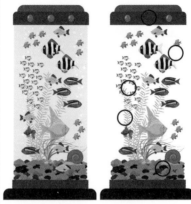

7. ODD ONE OUT
1 Mediterranean – the only sea, the rest are oceans.
2 Bronze – the only alloy, the rest are chemical elements.
3 Strawberry – the only red item, the rest are all yellow.
4 Sphynx – the only cat, the rest are all breeds of dog.
5 Venezuela – the only country in the northern hemisphere, the rest are all in the southern hemisphere.

76–77 SPATIAL VISUALIZATION

1. PYRAMID NETS
Two of the nets can be folded to make a complete 4-sided pyramid:

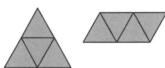

2. PAPER CUTTING
To make the shape pictured, make these three folds followed by this cut:

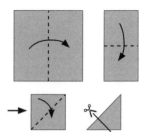

3. CUBE NETS
These three nets would not make cubes:

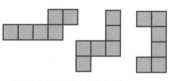

4. CUBE NET PATTERN
Cube net C.

5. CUBE VIEW

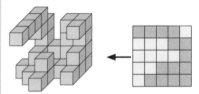

6. ROTATED CUBES
D is the odd one out–it has been reflected relative to the other three.

7. ROUTE MASTER
Instructions 3 result in the solid route that travels to the central house. Instructions 1 (dashed route) and 2 (dotted route) reach the holes shown.

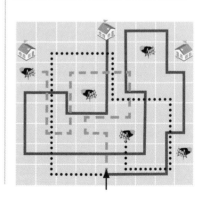

CHAPTER 4

84–85 MEMORY CHALLENGES

CHALLENGE 3: SUM MEMORY
1. EASY Set 1: 13 (=6+7)
Set 2: 19 (=7+12), 33 (=7+12+14)
2. MEDIUM
Set 1: 57 (=25+32), 53 (=21+32)
Set 2: 69 (=21+48)
3. HARD
Set 1: 97 (=17+80), 122 (=17+50+55)
Set 2: 180 (=49+52+79), 128 (=49+79),
101 (=49+52)

92–93 TRY NUMBER PUZZLES

CHALLENGE 1: NUMBER PYRAMIDS

1. EASY

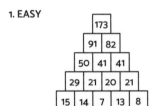

2. MEDIUM

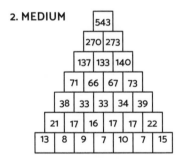

3. HARD

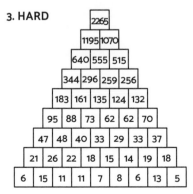

CHALLENGE 2: DIAGONAL TOTALS

1. EASY

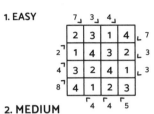

2. MEDIUM

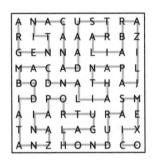

3. HARD

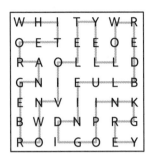

94–95 TRY WORD PUZZLES

CHALLENGE 1: LETTER SOUP
1. EASY Sports:
FOOTBALL, GOLF, TENNIS
2. MEDIUM Animals:
BEAR, CAMEL, GOAT, HORSE, TIGER
3. HARD Chemical elements:
CARBON, COPPER, GOLD,
HYDROGEN, MERCURY, SILICON

CHALLENGE 2: PATHFINDER
1. EASY Colors: WHITE, ORANGE,
BROWN, VIOLET, YELLOW, RED,
BLUE, INDIGO, PINK, GRAY

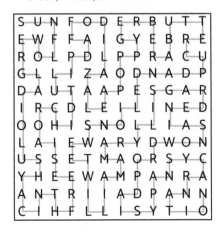

2. MEDIUM Countries: ARGENTINA,
CANADA, AUSTRALIA, BRAZIL, JAPAN,
THAILAND, CAMBODIA, TANZANIA,
PORTUGAL, HONDURAS, MEXICO

3. HARD Flowers: SUNFLOWER,
GLADIOLUS, HYACINTH, FREESIA,
ORCHID, TULIP, DAFFODIL, AZALEA,
POPPY, GERBERA, BUTTERCUP,
DANDELION, SWEET WILLIAM,
AMARYLLIS, GARDENIA, SNOWDROP,
DAISY, PANSY, CARNATION

CHALLENGE 1: ODD CUBE OUT
1. **EASY** Cube C
2. **MEDIUM** Cube C
3. **HARD** Cube D

CHALLENGE 2: VISUAL TRANSFORMATION
1. **EASY** B: Circles and lines are copied, then circles joined to two lines are shaded deeper purple, circles not joined to any lines have a "+" added inside.
2. **MEDIUM** C: The image is reflected horizontally, then the inner circles move to be on the intersection of two lines next to a solid circle, or they move horizontally to overlap the nearest single line next to a half-shaded circle.
3. **HARD** C: 1 deeply shaded square is drawn next to every triangle, 2 deeply shaded squares are heading away from every circle, and 3 deeply shaded squares are heading away from every star.

98–99 TRY LOGIC PUZZLES

CHALLENGE 1: SUDOKU

1. EASY

9	4	1	6	5	2	7	3	8
8	3	5	7	4	1	9	2	6
7	6	2	3	9	8	4	1	5
5	7	6	1	8	9	3	4	2
4	9	3	2	7	6	8	5	1
2	1	8	5	3	4	6	7	9
1	8	7	9	2	3	5	6	4
6	5	4	8	1	7	2	9	3
3	2	9	4	6	5	1	8	7

2. MEDIUM

4	2	9	7	8	3	6	1	5
5	8	7	4	6	1	2	3	9
3	1	6	2	5	9	8	4	7
6	5	4	8	9	2	1	7	3
9	3	8	5	1	7	4	6	2
2	7	1	3	4	6	9	5	8
8	4	3	1	2	5	7	9	6
1	9	5	6	7	8	3	2	4
7	6	2	9	3	4	5	8	1

3. HARD

5	6	4	3	1	9	8	7	2
8	9	1	5	2	7	6	4	3
7	3	2	4	6	8	5	1	9
6	1	3	8	5	2	7	9	4
9	7	8	1	3	4	2	5	6
2	4	5	7	9	6	3	8	1
4	2	6	9	8	5	1	3	7
1	5	7	2	4	3	9	6	8
3	8	9	6	7	1	4	2	5

CHALLENGE 2: OUTSIDE SUDOKU

1. EASY

```
          4              6
        9 2        8 3 3
        6 1        5 1 2        8
  4 | 8 3 4 9 6 1 2 7 5 | 5
    | 5 9 2 7 8 3 6 4 1 | 1
    | 7 6 1 2 5 4 3 9 8 | 3
  8 | 6 1 8 5 9 2 4 3 7 |
    | 4 2 3 1 7 8 5 6 9 | 5 6 9
    | 9 7 5 4 3 6 1 8 2 | 1
  4 | 1 4 9 3 2 7 8 5 6 |
6 2 | 2 5 6 8 4 9 7 1 3 |
  8 | 3 8 7 6 1 5 9 2 4 | 4 9
        3 4      6 1          1
        5               2          5
        8
```

2. MEDIUM

```
                  4
      5 6        3         2       7
      4 2        1 2       1       5
  4 | 4 6 8 1 7 9 2 3 5 | 2 5
    | 1 2 3 4 5 6 9 8 7 | 8
  7 | 5 9 7 3 2 8 1 4 6 | 1 6
    | 6 8 2 5 1 4 3 7 9 |
    | 9 4 1 7 6 3 5 2 8 | 5
7 5 | 7 3 5 9 8 2 4 6 1 | 1 4 6
  8 | 8 1 6 2 3 5 7 9 4 |
    | 3 5 9 6 4 7 8 1 2 | 1 2
7 4 | 2 7 4 8 9 1 6 5 3 | 3 6
        1 9       9 1      7        4
        7                  5
                           7
```

3. HARD

```
                  6                   9
      2 5 1    2 3         5 2 1
      | 6 5 1 2 7 9 4 3 8 | 8
7 3 2 | 2 7 3 1 4 8 5 6 9 |
      | 9 8 4 6 3 5 7 2 1 |
  3   | 3 4 7 5 1 2 8 9 6 | 6 8 9
  2   | 5 2 8 4 9 6 3 1 7 |
  9   | 1 6 9 7 8 3 2 4 5 | 4
  5   | 8 1 5 3 6 4 9 7 2 | 9
  2   | 7 3 2 9 5 1 6 8 4 | 4 6 8
  4   | 4 9 6 8 2 7 1 5 3 |
        4 3       9 6 1            4
        8 9             7
```

100–101 TRY CREATIVE REASONING PUZZLES

CHALLENGE 1: JIGSAW CUT

1. EASY

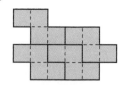

2. MEDIUM

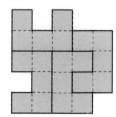

3. HARD

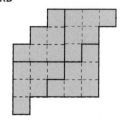

CHALLENGE 2: SNAKE

1. EASY

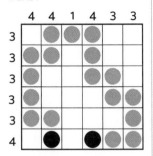

2. MEDIUM

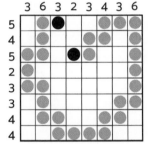

3. HARD

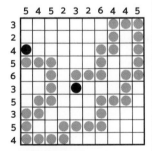

102–07 TRY MAKING MUSIC

EXERCISE 6: PITCH PERFECT

1 E	2 B	3 D
4 G	5 E	6 C
7 D	8 B	9 C
10 A	11 F	12 G
13 D	14 F	15 B
16 G	17 E	18 F
19 D	20 E	21 C
22 A		

EXERCISE 7: SHARPS AND FLATS

1 C-sharp	2 B-flat
3 G-flat	4 E-sharp
5 D-flat	6 E-flat
7 G-sharp	

120–23 TRY PLAYING CHESS

CHALLENGE 1: PAWN
You should queen your pawn by moving to square b8.

CHALLENGE 2: BISHOP
The bishop can move to seven squares and capture the black rook on square f6.

CHALLENGE 3: KNIGHT
The knight cannot capture any white pieces, but it can leap over the rook at f5 to capture the black rook at g5.

CHALLENGE 4: ROOK
The white rook should move from square a1 to a6 to e6 to e3 to c3 to c4.

CHALLENGE 5: QUEEN
The queen can safely capture the bishop on square d8.

CHALLENGE 6: KING
1. The white king cannot move to a safe square but the e4 bishop can capture the checking rook.

2. The white rook can block the check by moving to d1.

CHALLENGE 7: ACHIEVING CHECKMATE
• Moving the white queen to square f7 is checkmate, as the knight backs up the queen.
• Moving her to b8 allows the black king an escape to e7.
• Moving the queen to d8 can be blocked by the black knight moving to e8, but does lead to checkmate.
• Moving the white queen to c8 leads to disaster for white, as the black queen can then safely capture it.

148–51 TRY BIRDWATCHING

EXERCISE 2: PLUMAGE

A	Palm Warbler
B	Black-throated Green Warbler
C	Yellow-rumped Warbler
D	Hooded Warbler
E	Chestnut-sided Warbler
F	Kentucky Warbler
G	Blackburnian Warbler
H	Cape May Warbler
I	Canada Wabler

170–77 TRY A NEW LANGUAGE

EXERCISE 2: COUNT ON IT

33
ES treinta y tres
FR trente-trois
IT trentatré
DE dreiunddreißig
SV trettiotre

76
ES setenta y seis
FR soixante-seize
IT settantasei
DE sechsundsiebzig
SV sjuttiosex

95
ES noventa y cinco
FR quatre-vingt-quinze
IT novantacinque
DE fünfundneunzig
SV nittiofem

121
ES ciento veintiuno
FR cent vingt-et-un
IT centoventuno
DE einhunderteinundzwanzig
SV etthundratjugoett

374
ES trescientos setenta y cuatro
FR trois cent soixante-quatorze
IT trecentosettantaquattro
DE drehundertvierundsiebzig
SV trehundrasjuttiofyra

618
ES seiscientos diechiocho
FR six cent dix-huit
IT seicentodiciotto
DE sechshundertachtzehn
SV sexhundraarton

853
ES ochocientos cinquenta y tres
FR huit cent cinquante-trois
IT ottocentocinquantatré
DE achthundertdreiund-fünfzig
SV åttohundrafemtiotre

1,259
ES mil doscientos cincuenta y nueve
FR mille deux cent cinquante-neuf
IT milleduecentocinquanta-nove
DE eintausendzweihundert-neunundfünfzig
SV ettusen tvåhundrafemtio-nio

2,763
ES dos mil setecientos sesenta y tres
FR deux mille sept cent soixante-trois
IT duemilasettecento-sessantatré
DE zweitausendsieben-hundertdreiundsechzig
SV tvåtusen sjuhundra-sextiotre

INDEX

ACKNOWLEDGMENTS

Dorling Kindersley would like to thank the following people for their assistance in preparing this book: Alan Gow, professor of psychology at The Ageing Lab at Herriot-Watt University, Edinburgh, Scotland, for his advice and assistance in developing the contents; Clare Joyce for design assistance, Gillian Northcott Liles for the index, and Richard Gilbert for proofreading.

DK India would like to thank Priyal Mote for assistance in illustration and Vagisha Pushp for assistance in picture research.

The publisher would like to thank the following for their kind permission to reproduce their photographs:

(Key: a-above; b-below/bottom; c-centre; f-far; l-left; r-right; t-top)

123RF.com: Davor Dopar 157br, Rawpixel 143br, Liubou Yasiukovich 64tc; **Alamy Stock Photo:** Tommaso Altamura 38br, Wu Kailiang133clb, Roman Lacheev 163bc, Dale O'Dell 166br, Tetra Images, LLC 163br, Westend61 GmbH / Zerocreatives 104br; **Dorling Kindersley:** NASA 155clb, Jake Spicer 118ca, 118ca (main image), 118cra, 118cr, 118crb, 118br, 119cla, 119ca, 119ca (step 5); **Dreamstime.com:** Atoss1 47cl (mint), Katarzyna Bialasiewicz 133c, John Bjerk 133crb, Blueringmedia 64cb, Blueringmedia 71bl, Blueringmedia 31clb, Blueringmedia 44cra, 44clb, Kong Xiang Chen 145br, Peter Cripps 124bl, Dim154 161cra, Peter Hermes Furian 59t, Eric Gevaert 47fclb, Richard Jemmett 118cl, Khunaspix 142cr, Kateryna Khyzhniak 123bl, Ilga Lasmane 47fcl, Macrovector 48cr, 71cr, 81cla, Macrovector 75crb, 184ca, Macrovector 43c (Medicine bottles), Macrovector 44cla, Macrovector 4tr, 48clb, 81cl, Macrovector 80cra, Macrovector 80crb, 80br, Macrovector 81cb, 178cb, Macrovector 83cr, Macrovector 178bc (Tv), Macrovector 178bc, Macrovector 178c, Sergiy1975 112cla, Kamil Sulun 99cr, Alena Valodzkina 47cl, Verdateo 106bc, Veruska1969 133fclb, Wirestock 137bl; **Fotolia:** Thomas Dobner / Dual Aspect 148crb; **Getty Images:** 10'000 Hours / DigitalVision 31tr, Luis Alvarez / DigitalVision 36ca, Thomas Barwick / DigitalVision 123br, Thomas Barwick / DigitalVision 156br, Thomas Barwick / Stone 169br, Boston Globe / Contributor 159ca, DigitalVision / Jon Feingersh Photography Inc 46cb, DigitalVision / MoMo Productions 6br, DigitalVision / The Good Brigade 6cr, E+ / katleho Seisa 175br, E+ / wilpunt 47clb, EyeEm / Phongthorn Hiranlikhit 47ca, Rana Faure / Corbis / VCG 119br, John Fedele 38clb, Halfpoint Images / Moment 34, David Jakle 6cl, Jetta Productions Inc / DigitalVision 141br, JGI / Jamie Grill 95tr, Jose Luis Pelaez Inc / DigitalVision 83cla, Mint Images RF 167tr, Kelvin Murray / Stone 81tr, Nico De Pasquale Photography / Moment 113tr, Photographer's Choice RF / Stuart Minzey 47clb (Star anise), Mike Raabe / The Image Bank 160br, Marc Romanelli 146bl, Christianto Soning / EyeEm 155bc, Stone / Thomas Barwick 6tl, 6tr, UpperCut Images 46fcrb; **Getty Images / iStock:** 4x6 156c, 156bc, 157c, 157cr, 157cb, 157crb, AIS60 129bl, DragonImages 42cra, E+ / lisegagne 6bl, E+ / Nikola Ilic 136tr, E+ / valentinrussanov 6bc, Sam Edwards / OJO Images 159c, FatCamera 159cra, Fstop123 151br, Kali9 / E+ 144cl, Tarik Kizilkaya 169bl, Klubovy 161br, Kohei_Hara / E+ 117bl, Olivier Laurent 105tr, Martinns / E+ 45bl, Terdpong Pangwong 68bl, PeopleImages / E+ 120crb, RgStudio / E+ 162br, Senya211 133cb, slavikbig 134br, SolidMaks 151cr, Stockbyte / Visage 6c, SurfUpVector 39ca, Thurtell 159tr, Tomwang112 35tl, Uthenism 31cla, Val_Th / Istock Editorial 106br, Tero Vesalainen 111br, Vgajic / E+ 128br, Vladimir Vladimirov / E+ 109tr, Warrengoldswain 131bl; **Anderson Diego Lopes:** 141bl; **NASA:** GSFC / Arizona State University 155crb; **naturepl.com:** Loic Poidevin 151tr; Science Photo Library: Eye Of Science 17br, Alfred Pasieka 22cb, Alfred Pasieka 22crb, Alain Pol, ISM 12bl; **Shutterstock.com:** Africa Studio 47cla, Jane Kelly 39crb, 82cb, McLittle Stock 126bc, Rawpixel.com 36br; **Wellcome Collection:** Dr Flavio Dell'Acqua 14

All other images © Dorling Kindersley
For further information see: www.dkimages.com